What the Experts are Saying About
The Take Charge Beauty Book
and Natural Hair and Skin Care Products

"This is the most innovative, honest and healthy beauty book I have ever read. *The Take Charge Beauty Book* is a work of art that shares the magic of natural products in a simple yet thorough way. The information is written in easy-to-understand language, and Aubrey and Susan even provide formulas for those adventurous types who wish to make their own natural cosmetics. *The Take Charge Beauty Book* is a magnificent coaching tool for anyone interested in the natural approach to inner and outer beauty success."

—Debbi Lawrence
USA Olympic Race Walker

"I've used Aubrey's products for me and my family for ten years. I use them because they are a wonderful mix of art and science, and that mix provides beautiful results with a very minimal risk of skin/scalp allergies and irritations.... There's always some art and folklore involved in choosing combinations of herbs that not only do the job, but look and smell attractive, and have synergy when blended. That only comes with trial and error, experience, and a real love and commitment to the design of herbal products. I don't see another major company in the natural products industry that goes as far in this direction as Aubrey's. Now this book tells you how to make natural products and how to use them." (See page 213.)

—C. Leigh Broadhurst, Ph.D.
Author, *Diabetes: Prevention and Cure* (Kensington Publishing, 1999).

"In Aubrey Hampton and Susan Hussey's, *The Take Charge Beauty Book*, Aubrey makes a tofu-based Essential Fatty Acid Cream Base (Formula #1). Unlike mineral oil cold creams that can stay on top of your skin and clog your pores, leaving a greasy residue, this cream base is absorbed rapidly, functioning as a carrying agent for herbs, vitamins and other nutrients. It increases absorption and soften and moisturizes the complexion. (I'd rather put tofu on my face than eat it anyhow.)

"Aubrey kindly names his new rosemary-sage shampoo for me, but for reasons other than I had intended. 1 was recommending lemon-balm, rosemary and sage shampoo for Alzheimer's, which Aubrey doesn't even mention or index. Serendipitously, 1 made the recommendation before I had learned of the pronounced choline-sparing (antialzheimerian) activity of peppermint, and even more serendipitously, Aubrey has peppermint as the lead ingredient in his new Formula #19, 'Dr. Duke's Hair Saver Rosemary and Sage Shampoo.' I think of it more as a brain saver than hair saver.

—James A. Duke, Ph.D.
Author, *The Green Pharmacy* (Rodale Press, 1997)
Botanical Consultant
Herbal Vineyard, Inc.

"Natural cosmetics, whether homemade or purchased from select national leaders in the natural product industry, avoid the toxic chemicals often inherent in mass produced cosmetics. Instead, they rely on herbal ingredients, combined with nutrients and other safe, natural substances that have a proven record of efficacy and safety. What's more, my own experience and that of my family and patients indicates that natural is better when it comes to looking and feeling your best." (See page 212.)

—David Steinman
Author, *Diet for a Poisoned Planet* (Ballantine, 1992)
The Safe Shopper's Bible, with Samuel S. Epstein, M.D. (Macmillan, 1995).

"As the author of a book that uncovered the dirty secrets of the cosmetic industry, I know firsthand that commercial cosmetic products may be loaded with chemical toxins that increase your risk for allergies, irritation, and even cancer. By learning the secrets of making your own natural cosmetics and personal care products, you'll not only save money and have fun making them, you'll be going a long way toward detoxifying your skin from the many unsafe chemicals in cosmetic products. Ginseng, biotin, mucopolysaccharides, coltsfoot, horsetail, yucca, quillaya bark, rosemary—these are the ingredients of safe and healthy beauty." (See page 213.)

Gary Wilkholm, M.D.
Editor, *The Doctors' Prescription for Healthy Living*

"The success of commercial cosmetics is based on the public's lack of knowledge about biology and chemistry. Madison Avenue, with all its tricks and glamour, can perpetuate the cosmetic industry indefinitely because people like to look good. With an impatient world of instant gratification, the long term effects of what we do to our bodies are not considered as serious consequences... You may not be able to control many of the pollutants around you, but now you can have control over what you put on your hair and skin, whether you make it yourself or have the knowledge of the best natural products to buy. Making and using these products is a win-win situation because they enhance your appearance, make you feel good about yourself, and are not harmful to you and the environment as are many of the commercial cosmetics, perfumes and sprays."

—Karla C. D. McNamara, M.D.

"Aubrey Hampton and Susan Hussey cover all the bases and provide a great deal of very useful and important information about natural skin and hair care treatments."

—Donald Charles Richardson
Author, http://TheGuysGuide.com

"When I have taken my treks through the rain forest in South America, sometimes leading groups of health care practitioners, natural personal care products is all I allow them to bring, and Aubrey's products lead the pack. Using natural hair and skin care products means that we're not just not polluting the environment, but we're also using something that is great for us.... My baby has only known natural products. My wife and I have used natural products for decades. We consciously feel so much better and happier, in our right stance with the planet, with the universe." (See page 214.)

—Marcus Laux, N.D.
Professor, College of Naturopathic Medicine, Portland, OR

"As a family health physician who also specializes in helping patients overcome both environmental and occupational chemical exposures, I'm very concerned about the types of consumer products that people bring into their homes. One area of particular concern is the cosmetics and personal care products that my patients pick up from the local drug and department stores.... I stress to my patients the health virtues of natural cosmetics, whether made at home or purchased from their local health food store. I'd much rather see my patients applying green tea and milk thistle to their skin than quaternium-15 or some other toxic compound!" (See page 211.)

—Megan Shields, M.D.

"I have been delighted with the natural products you will see in this book. I use natural products for myself and my patients, products that do not contain solvents such as propyl alcohol, propyl paraben, PVP, EDTA, benzene, toluene, etc... The public on a whole is unaware of how many people are sensitive to these solvents and the various synthetic chemicals in cosmetics. Being a naturopathic physician, I see this on a daily basis. Not only are these completely natural products healthy and safe, they really nourish the hair and skin."

—Victoria Zupa,
N.D.

"Four months ago my business manager introduced me to Aubrey's book *Natural Organic Hair and Skin Care*, and many of his natural products, For the last 17 years I have been committed to bringing the highest quality natural beauty and health care through the use of acupuncture and scientific nutrition. With great satisfaction I can highly recommend to my patients Aubrey and Susan's *The Take Charge Beauty Book* as the ultimate guide for hair and skin care."

—David J. Nickel, O.M.D.

"More and more people are becoming mindful of what goes into their bodies by reading food labels... and seeking more natural, organic foods and herbs. It's just as important to be aware of what goes *on* our bodies. *The Take Charge Beauty Book* is a comprehensive guide that will help you make the right cosmetic choices, with formulas for natural products that you can create yourself. The book gives you an alternative to chemical-laden cosmetics by helping you find, purchase and correctly use natural ingredients for your hair and skin."

—Gerrie E. Summers,
Beauty Editor, *Today's Black Woman*

"The skin is like a human sink which absorbs the toxins in commercial cosmetic and personal care products. I'm so concerned about this that I tell all my patients to always seek safe and healthy natural cosmetics. Sometimes I even show them myself how they can make a great conditioner for their hair simply by using the milk protein found in yogurt, or how they can create highlights in their hair with the use of certain safe herbal preparations, or how ginseng works as a scalp stimulant, and biotin actually helps to thicken the hair. There are all sorts of techniques and tricks that consumers can learn to make their own great cosmetics." (See page 212.)

—L. Stephen Coles, M.D., Ph.D., editor
The Journal of Anti-Aging Medicine

ACKNOWLEDGEMENTS

The authors wish to acknowledge the printers at Organica Press, Roland Gerke and Curtis Barrow; our graphic designer Sean Sanczel; our art director Carol Glass; the lovely Priscilla De Francesco for lending her face to the pages of our book and going through the facial exercises and step-by-step methods; all the fine people at Rose Printing; and of course, our editor Silvia Curbelo.

THE TAKE CHARGE BEAUTY BOOK

The Natural Guide to Beautiful Hair and Skin

By
Aubrey Hampton
&
Susan Hussey

Organica Press
4419 N. Manhattan Ave.
Tampa, FL 33614
www.organicanews.com

Published by
Organica Press
4419 N. Manhattan Ave.
Tampa, Florida 33614

First Edition

Hampton, Aubrey and Hussey, Susan
The Take Charge Beauty Book:
The Natural Guide to Beautiful Hair and Skin
Library of Congress Catalogue Card Number
98-068046
ISBN 0-939157-09-8

Disclaimer

No part of this book is intended for the treatment of disease, and neither the author nor publisher assumes any liability for such use. Readers with skin conditions or other ailments should seek competent medical advice. The descriptions herein of products or substances are for educational purposes only and are not intended as recommendations by the author or publisher. The use of any product or substance discussed in this book rests on the judgment of the reader. The authors are not responsible for any allergic reactions due to the use of any product in this book. A 24-hour patch test is recommended. All formulas and cosmetic products are for external use only.

Trademark Notice

Because a portion of this book describes and comments on various cosmetic ingredients, some such products or ingredients are identified by their trade names. In most cases, these designations are claimed as legally protected trademarks by the companies that make or package the products or ingredients, and where such designation exists, it is for reference only. It is not our intent to use any of these names generically, and the reader is cautioned to investigate a claimed trademark before using it for any purpose except to refer to the product to which it is attached and for personal use. The manufacturing of the formulas for commercial distribution is strictly forbidden. Some products or ingredients are legally protected by trademarks and permission must be obtained from the trademark holders (or contact the authors and/or publisher).

Table of Contents

How This Book Came About

Aubrey Hampton has been creating natural cosmetics under his brand name of Aubrey Organics® for over 30 years, and his hair and skin care products are recognized and sold all over the world. His is a story of the little fish in the big pond of the cosmetic industry, of a man beating the odds and making waves by manufacturing and selling all-natural cosmetics on his own terms.

Aubrey's connection to natural ingredients and natural products goes way back to his roots in rural Indiana. Born of French parents, Aubrey's mother was an herbalist and small time entrepreneur who created her own beauty products from scratch during the Depression, generating a little extra income for her family by selling them to friends and neighbors in hand-labeled glass bottles that read "Made by Marguerite."

Her days in that sunny kitchen were filled with jars and vials of golden oils and powders, and handwritten recipes she adapted again and again as she tried new ways to put ingredients together. Guided by Aubrey's father, a union organizer and part-time organic farmer, she grew many of her own herbs organically and learned to use them in her preparations. As Marguerite's homemade soaps and creams gained in popularity and the demand grew, she needed an extra pair of hands, so she trained nine-year-old Aubrey to help out in the kitchen.

He was neat and exacting and seldom spilled things, measuring herbs in little wads of paper he weighed on a scale, and stirring thick batches of her homemade cream base that smelled of dried flowers and freshly turned earth. These were the green, pungent smells of his childhood, smells that are as comforting today as that faraway kitchen of his youth. A high point was traveling to Louisville to visit the pharmacy where his mother bought supplies, standing around surrounded by the many vials of essential oils—lavender, rosemary, sage, and especially, fragrant eucalyptus, from which Marguerite made a bar soap young Aubrey would painstakingly pour into little wooden molds to let harden.

By age 18, Aubrey set out to pursue a very different dream—to work in the theatre. He did the only thing that made sense then—he moved to New York City to study acting. Eventually, though, he switched gears, obtaining a Ph.D. in organic chemistry from New York University while working his way through school. His thesis on the effects of glycogen on the skin would be instrumental in the creation of one of Aubrey Organics® earliest and most successful natural products, GPB (Glycogen Protein Balancer) Hair Conditioner and Nutrient. But first Aubrey would get some experience under his belt working for the cosmetic industry, including a six-year stint at Fabergé, where he learned more than he ever wanted to know about the manufacture and marketing of mass-produced beauty products.

In 1967, while recovering from a serious automobile accident that injured his neck, he sought relief from troublesome aches and pains by returning to familiar ground. Using the skills he had learned from his mother, he began work-ing on a therapeutic bath treatment to help ease stiffness and muscle strain. Into a coconut oil soap base he blended peppermint, a natural anti-inflammatory, rose-mary and sage, excellent skin toners, and that old childhood favorite, eucalyptus oil. At the urging of macrobiotic guru George Oshawa, whose East Village café Aubrey frequented in the 1960s, he put in wild ginger, not the extract but the actual ground root, for greater potency. The result was Relax-R-Bath, the first Aubrey Organics® product which, more than 30 years later, is still a top-seller.

Aubrey is fond of saying that his secret is, "No secret—just read my labels!" More than 30 years later, he still makes products the way his mother made hers. Heading a multimillion dollar, multinational company, Aubrey still creates every formula that bears his name and personally oversees the way his products are manufactured—by hand, in small batches, and using the finest all-natural ingre-dients available, organically grown ones whenever possible.

Susan Hussey joined Aubrey Organics® in 1984, a graduate student in En-glish literature trying to earn some extra money typing invoices for the main office. Her literary background soon came in handy. Aubrey had just completed the manuscript of his first book, *Natural Organic Hair and Skin Care*, and Susan was promptly hired on as editor. (Published in 1987 by Aubrey's own publishing house, Organica Press, the book is now in its seventh reprint and still going strong.) Today Susan is Vice-President of Marketing and International Sales, and is cred-ited for introducing Aubrey Organics® products into many world markets, includ-ing Japan, Korea, Taiwan, Portugal, Canada, Puerto Rico and Germany.

Susan's interest in natural products can also be traced back to her early home life, though for very different reasons. Her mother was a 21-year survivor of the new "kidney machine," the first woman in Indiana to be put on home dialysis. Living with the consequences of her mother's long, difficult illness taught her early the importance of caring for one's health. As a teenager Susan began read-ing about nutritional healing and shopping in health food stores.

It was not a direct path to her final destination as a top executive in a company known for its ethical, earth-friendly products. Susan joined a small Canadian circus as a magician's assistant, appearing nightly in the center ring to be sawed in half or be made to disappear into thin air. It was a startling change, one that forced her to reevaluate her former, no-makeup "pseudointellectual-hippie-chick" look. She found herself facing a nightly audience and having to look present-able—downright glamorous even. Like most women searching for ways to en-hance their appearance, Susan turned to cosmetics for a little help. Early on she had learned to read ingredients labels, and now she was shocked to find most beauty aids displaying several inches of chemical-sounding names on their bottles and jars, each more unpronounceable than the last.

Eventually, she stopped buying and using synthetic beauty products and be-gan making her own masks at home from ingredients purchased at the health food store. Every night she rinsed her face with a skin-clearing blend of warm water and cider vinegar. "I smelled like a pickle," she says, "but my complexion looked great!"

The Take Charge Beauty Book

Whether her walking into the Aubrey Organics® offices as a temp worker all those years ago was a question of karma, or just a stroke of good luck, Aubrey and Susan's long and very special working relationship was well on its way. Through the years Susan helped Aubrey launch and promote many successful hair and skin care products, and edited *Organica*, Aubrey's quarterly newspaper on activism and the arts. They even produced plays together at their jointly operated Gorilla Theatre in Tampa, Florida. But they had never really considered writing a book together.

The idea surfaced during a promotional tour of Aubrey's latest book, *What's in Your Cosmetics?* (Odonian Press, 1995). They had set up personal appearances in a number of bookstores and health food stores nationwide. To help liven things up, they cooked up the idea of a hands-on demonstration Aubrey could do during his talks. Right on the spot, he would create a hand lotion from simple ingredients stirred together and invite audience members to come up and try a little on their skin. It was a great crowd pleaser, and it worked particularly well on TV talk shows.

At book signings people began coming up to Aubrey not only to congratulate him on the new book, but to inquire about the next one, the one containing the wonderful hand lotion recipe he had created moments before during his presentation.

It was an idea whose time had come, Susan and Aubrey were certain. What if women, tired of chemical brews and overpriced, overhyped beauty potions-of-the-week could actually open their refrigerators and their cupboards and make their own beauty products from scratch, just like Marguerite did in her farmhouse kitchen, just like Susan did at the tiny sink of that pint-sized circus trailer? Say, a skin-revitalizing mask of organic tomatoes, yogurt and bilberry extract? Or a moisturizer made from silken tofu, aloe vera and dried green barley? But recipes do not a great beauty book make: how about which natural hair and skin care products are really natural, and where to buy them, and what ingredients to avoid? Plus, what are the best choices women can make in their diet, nutritional supplements and exercise that will result in healthier and more beautiful skin and hair? The possibilities were endless. And no one was more suited for the challenge than these two unconventional souls who had already made their very visible mark in the cosmetic industry.

– Silvia Curbelo
Editor
Organica Press

3

Introduction

T his is a take charge book. It is designed to help you regain and maintain control of how you take care of your hair and skin—from what you put *on* your body to what you put in it. These pages will challenge you to bypass all the media hype and miracle potions and offer you sensible ways to be beautiful on your own terms.

This book may very well be the cosmetic industry's greatest nightmare. It will empower you to set aside all sorts of expensive, synthetically produced, elaborately packaged beauty aids with millions of dollars of advertising behind them and show you how to create completely natural products right in your own kitchen, products made with ingredients you control—that come from nature and are more compatible with your living body. Also, it will inform you of what to look for in the products you buy off the shelf so that you are choosing with your best health in mind.

Let's consider all the chemicals that come in contact with your body in just the first few minutes of every day. Rubbing your eyes, you climb out of bed and stumble into the bathroom. First you might reach for your favorite toothpaste. That bright red color certainly didn't come from nature! Stepping into the shower you notice the bottle of bright green shampoo, so thick a pearl takes a whole minute to fall through it. Right beside it is that tube of conditioner—the one that smells like a rain forest, if such a thing is possible. You pick up the soap to wash your face—a bar so pure it floats, they say, so it must be good for you.

Seated at your dressing table, it's time to get your face ready to greet the day. You open the jar of that moisturizer your mother recommended now that you're not as young as you used to be—but why does it make your skin look greasy and feel dry at the same time? The liquid makeup you bought at the department store should take care of any spots and imperfections, or maybe cover up those few lines that have begun to develop. Now a spot of eyeliner and a dash of that new lipstick they're advertising everywhere, the kind that won't wipe off no matter how hard you rub your lips. It was expensive enough, but if you want the best, you have to pay for it, right?

Well, not exactly.

If this is how you start your day, you've quite possibly come in contact with over 100 chemicals already, and you haven't even left your bathroom yet! You can rest assured you will be exposed to hundreds—maybe thousands—more throughout your day. The Worldwatch Institute states that some 75,000 chemicals have the potential of coming in contact with our bodies at any given time. And you can be sure none of them were developed with your health in mind.

Let's face it, we live in a vast chemical soup. Everything from the air we breathe to the water we drink to the food we eat is tainted with man-made substances that can wreak havoc on our bodies and cause a variety of ills, from mild allergic reactions to cancer!

Today many of us already shop in health food stores to help minimize our exposure to these chemicals. We drink bottled water. We buy organic produce to avoid ingesting dangerous pesticides with our carrots and beets, and buy hormone- and antibiotic-free poultry and beef. We've even trained ourselves to read labels and avoid certain synthetic preservatives, colors and flavoring agents in favor of more natural, minimally processed ingredients. Finally, we are learning to take steps to help control what goes into our bodies. But what about what goes *on* our bodies—on our skin, hair and scalp?

The Chemical Question

In the 19th century three trends changed the quality of cosmetics: 1) doctors and medical personnel stopped manufacturing, prescribing and promoting beauty creams and lotions, leaving the field open to entrepreneurs; 2) consumer services dealing in beauty prospered, thus the proliferation of aestheticians, hair salons and spas; 3) the chemical industry began creating petrochemicals and other synthetic chemicals which would be widely used in cosmetic preparations. Of these, the third is by far the most important—and the most devastating—in terms of our health and the health of the planet.

Decades ago we were quick to embrace new synthetic chemicals because they brought with them the promise of a brighter, more efficient future. But we know now that the millions of gallons of fossil fuels we burn every day (coal, oil, gas) are profoundly changing our air, food, water, indeed, every inch of our existence. Today petrochemicals are found in everything from clothing, bedding, rugs, furniture and draperies to perfumes, pesticides, cleaners, waxes, printers' inks, paints, solvents, toothpastes, mouthwashes, hair sprays, shampoos, lotions, drugs, and last but not least, artificial colors and preservatives that end up in many of the products we use, including the very foods we eat.

Compared to natural substances that have been in use for thousands of years, these man-made substances are relatively new to us. They have been around for only a short time, and their full effect on the human body has not yet been established. It could be decades, even hundreds of years, before we understand the consequences of long-term exposure to many—if not all—synthetic chemicals.

In the face of overwhelming evidence that many synthetic chemicals are harmful, it's best to take the high road and live by a simple premise: Anything you put on your skin will get *under* your skin. So why put anything on your skin you wouldn't dream of putting into your mouth?

It is a matter of common sense that natural substances are more compatible with our living tissues. Victoria Zupa, N.D., a highly respected naturopath from Darien, Connecticut, says, "The public at large is unaware of how many people are sensitive to solvents and other synthetic chemicals. Being a naturopathic physician, I see this on a daily basis. Not only are natural products healthy and safe, they really nourish the hair and skin. To eliminate toxic solvents and other synthetic chemicals from commercial usage is a great benefit to all mankind."

Perhaps Dr. Marcus Laux, N.D., sums it up best: "There is no doubt in my mind that whatever touches your skin ends up in your body. It can help you or hurt you. I have found that natural hair and skin care products—when they are truly natural—feel better on the skin, and cause fewer problems." (See Part VI, "What to Look for, What to Avoid in Your Cosmetic Products.")

Cosmetics, the Cosmos and You

Since the beginning, long before recorded history, beauty has been paramount in people's lives. Then as now, beauty has been a sign of success, of power, and many women and men will do—or pay—anything to achieve it. From the ancient Chinese practice of foot binding to the more modern techniques of liposuction and silicone implants, examples of the lengths people—women in particular—resort to in their search for beauty are plentiful, ranging from the bizarre to the downright tragic. For thousands of years women have blinded themselves with eyelash dyes, painted their skin with lead to make it appear whiter (dying from lead poisoning in the process) and dramatically increased their chances of developing cancer with synthetic hair dyes.

The word cosmetic comes from the Greek *kosmein*, which means "to arrange," and from *kosmos*, a concept discussed by Greek philosopher Pythagoras in 550 B.C., and defined by *The American Heritage Dictionary* as "the universe regarded as a harmonious whole."

To the ancient Greeks, being physically beautiful was being in harmony with the universe, thus one's own physical beauty was representative of the "cosmos" in miniature. We don't generally think of cosmetics in such heady terms, but if we understand the intimate relationship between one's appearance and the idea of harmony—of balance within nature—we might come to understand how important it is to feel good about the way we look in terms of our physical and emotional well being. Having beautiful hair and skin puts us in harmony with the universe, and using all-natural substances towards this end helps restore a natural balance within our bodies, and contributes greatly to our personal health and peace of mind.

Taking Charge of Your Hair and Skin

If you read the ingredients labels of all the various commercial cosmetic brands and compare them, you will actually find very little difference between them. In label after label, right below the same flowery, friendly-sounding copy promising a more radiant and beautiful you, you'll come across the same old list of synthetic chemicals. The same petrochemicals, synthetic preservatives, emulsifiers and foam builders, the same artificial colors and fragrances will be there, with only slight variations—a drop or two of this or that "natural" herb, often used in quantities so small, it is hard to imagine what effect it could have on your skin or hair.

Not only are most of these cosmetics a waste of time and money, but many of them can do far more harm than good. Here's a little known fact: It is not unusual to find that what mass manufacturers spend on the ingredients in one of their cosmetics can be as little as one-hundredth of the cost of the finished product! That means as little as one cent out of every dollar you spend on that high end jar of cream from your department store has gone towards the contents of that cream. The rest goes towards packaging (that lovely frosted glass bottle), promoting (that "free" tote bag with each $25 purchase), advertising (those dreamy TV ads) and distributing the product from Paris to Peoria. That should tell you something about the priorities of cosmetic manufacturers, an industry estimated by Solomon Brothers at $55 billion in 1997.

Every day we become more and more aware that the chemicalization of our earth is having disastrous, long-range effects on the ecological balance of our planet. Yet, we still have a long way to go to make bottom-line-driven cosmetic manufacturers more responsible about what goes into their creams and lotions.

Cosmetics are the least regulated products under the Federal Food, Drug and Cosmetic Act, and nothing protects the consumer from misrepresentation by companies claiming their products are natural. Some manufacturers take the view that as long as there's a drop or two of something natural in a product, that product is natural, no matter how synthetic the formula happens to be. A few years ago one so-called "natural" cosmetic company went as far as to run a series of ads educating the public to the "fact" that natural substances actually work better with synthetic chemicals in them!

A Note About our Recipes

The recipes in this book are based on ancient herbal traditions from around the world. They are made with herbs, plant extracts and other ingredients proven safe by thousands of years of human use, natural substances that were around long before petrochemicals entered the picture, before synthetic preservatives colors or fragrances made their all-too-disturbing mark.

You can purchase these natural ingredients right in your local health food store, or buy them through natural products mail order catalogs. Some of these ingredients can even be found in your supermarket, but read the labels to make sure they have not been "enhanced" or preserved with artificial colors or synthetic preservatives.

You will be surprised at the quality of the cosmetics you can make in your own kitchen, products that are fresher, better and less expensive than store bought ones. You will also find many of the same ingredients you used to create a facial moisturizer will turn up later in a recipe for a hair conditioner or a liquid soap. Once you've made the initial investment, purchasing many of these herbs, vitamins and essential oils, you'll be able to use them over and over to make your own beauty aids at a fraction of the cost.

– Aubrey Hampton
– Susan Hussey
New York City, 2000

How to Use This Book

This book is broken down into seven sections, arranged for easy access. Part I will tell you all about your skin—how it works and what it needs to stay healthy. In this section Susan will show you exactly how to do a complete Natural Method facial (using the products you make, of course), how to give yourself a facial massage, how to do an acupressure "face lift," and other special beauty treatments for your complexion.

Part II deals with the structure and function of your hair, and how our Natural Method of hair care can make it fuller, lustrous and more manageable from the very first time you try it.

In Part III Susan takes you through the many different kinds of supplements available in your health food store and what their value is to your skin, hair and body.

Part IV is a close-up view of all the ingredients you'll need to make your natural cosmetics, why Aubrey chose them and why they are important to the health of your hair and skin.

Part V is the heart of the book, Aubrey's 30 natural cosmetic formulas that are going to change your life. We call these "gourmet cosmetics" because they're the best you will find anywhere at any price.

Part VI is what we call our cosmetics hit-list. It tells you what to look for in commercial cosmetic preparations, and what synthetic ingredients you should avoid. Be sure to take this list with you when you go shopping for cosmetics—it could spare you rashes and other potentially serious allergic reactions. Don't leave home without it!

Part VII is our natural resources section. It not only lists all the ingredients featured in our formulas, but also gives you a list of preferred brands to make your shopping easier.

Part VIII is our list of recommended natural cosmetics you can buy. It's our own list, which means we've tried these products. This doesn't mean you have to buy them.

We hope you put this book to work for you. In doing so, you will gain a new understanding and appreciation for your body, your environment and the earth we live in.

15 Common Cosmetic Myths

1. Cosmetics can make you look young again.

If a product claims to take 20 years off your face and make wrinkles disappear, read the label. What magic ingredients will you find there that will actually make lines and imperfections vanish and bring youth back to your skin again? Chances are what you'll see is not some rare component from the fountain of youth, but a list of petrochemicals and other synthetics as long as your arm. The truth is no cosmetic can turn back the clock and make your skin look and feel, at age 40 or 50, the way it did at 20. Staying young requires much more than slathering on some expensive cream once a day. It is a committed strategy of diet, hair and skin care, exercise, and even attitude. Everything counts, and the earlier you start, the better! In this book you will learn about certain herbals that, when applied topically, actually help your body rebuild the collagen in your skin and help it retain moisture and elasticity—the two things that keep skin looking young. You will discover what vitamins and food supplements work best to promote lustrous, healthy hair and a more youthful complexion. While no cosmetic manufacturer can honestly claim to take away wrinkles, we can guarantee that using high quality cosmetics made from completely natural sources is an important step in keeping your skin healthy, clear and youthful.

2. Price makes a difference.

"It's more expensive, therefore it's better" seems to be the motto of the salespeople at the cosmetic counter of your local department store. This makes sense in theory, and it gives them an opportunity to justify the outrageous price tags on some of these high end creams and lotions. Here is one sad fact: The main difference between an expensive cosmetic and an inexpensive one is the price of the packaging and the size of the cosmetic manufacturer's advertising budget, not what's *in* the bottle. If you're not convinced, compare the ingredients of an inexpensive moisturizer or facial toner from a discount store with its department store counterpart. Chances are there won't be much difference.

Remember: cosmetic companies are in the business of selling dreams and spinning myths, and that, in part, is what you pay for. Here's an example of the cosmetic industry at work: In the early 1980s a big name cosmetic company promised that their new "cellular repair cream" would make wrinkles disappear and literally take away years from your face. This latest magic potion used actual cells from a certain species of black sheep. These cells, the story goes, would go into your skin and instantly replace your aging cells. A tiny bottle of this amazing cream sold for more than $50. Soon other cosmetic manufacturers jumped on the band wagon with their dead sheep cells. By the early 1990s—ten years, several hundred dollars and a lot of dead sheep later—the people who faithfully used this cream looked, well, ten years older! Don't buy a claim like this, and don't waste your money.

3. There *are* magic ingredients.

Leave the magic tricks to the magicians and illusionists. In the world of cosmetics, there are no magic potions. This is not to say that some herbals and other nutrients don't do wonders for your skin and hair. But the amounts of these herbals included in mass-produced cosmetics are probably insufficient to do much good for you. The real trick is to learn what natural ingredients will work best to restore health and beauty to your hair and skin, and then use them in your own cosmetic formulas.

4. There is a European or Asian or Himalayan mystique.

Another buzz word in the early 1980s (a big time for the cosmetic industry) was "Swiss collagen." The widely circulated story was that this ingredient would wipe away wrinkles and replenish your "cross-linked" collagen. Even a famous heart surgeon got behind the magic "Swiss collagen" youth-reviving face cream. People bought it for high prices. Nobody asked the question: Does collagen have a nationality? Why is Swiss collagen superior to, say, Mexican collagen, or South African collagen? This is an example of what in the industry is known as the "European mystique." Sure enough, there even was a "European Collagen Formula" on the market! Better cosmetics do not necessarily come from Europe—or any other part of the world for that matter— although where a product is made can affect *how* that product is made and what it contains. Some of the supposedly "natural cosmetics" from Europe, for example, have just as many synthetic chemicals in them as any American brand. There is no European mystique; there is no "secret formula" from the Himalayas, and there is no "miracle cream" made by an ancient sage living in a tiny village who gave it in strictest confidence to us, so that we could turn around and sell it to you for an outrageous but justifiable price. The fact is, no area of the world has an exclusive corner on making products that guarantee younger-looking skin and fuller hair.

5. What I put on my skin is not as important as what I put into my body.

That's what some people may lead you to believe, but it simply isn't true. The fact is that anything you put on your skin will end up *in* your body within minutes. Our chapter on the skin deals at length with some absorption issues, and later on we offer a list of commonly used chemicals you should avoid putting on your skin and scalp. The good news is that, in the same way that the skin can absorb harmful substances that eventually make their way into vital organs of the body, the skin can also take in beneficial substances, such as herbals, vitamins and other nutrients. One of the major purposes of this book is to take a new look at beauty and health from the outside in—what to let into your body, and what to keep out at all costs.

6. Natural ingredients need synthetic ingredients to work better.

This myth is an odd one, because the truth is exactly the opposite: natural ingredients work best when there are NO synthetic additives in the formula. A large, so-called "natural" cosmetic manufacturer got behind this one in a big way and actually ran ads explaining why they used some synthetic ingredients in many of their products. Rationalization goes a long way, but it doesn't change the facts. A little natural is good, but *100% natural* is as good as it gets!

7. Natural ingredients can be dangerous for your skin and hair.

This is quite a spin, indeed, and is a more extreme variation of the previous myth. Cosmetic manufacturers put the most awful chemical additives in their products—formaldehyde, mineral oil, artificial colors made with coal tar and other petrochemicals—then they turn around and warn you that natural ingredients can be dangerous. This is an obvious scare tactic to make you worry about natural ingredients and accept their way of doing things (synthetically). Most natural poisons, such as strychnine and arsenic, have been around for thousands of years, and we know to avoid them. On the other hand, the myriad chemicals mass produced cosmetics contain have only been around for a handful of years, and we don't really know what longterm effects they'll have on our bodies. Thousands of years of human use have established herbals as safe and effective. We know far more about them than we do the man-made chemicals that have been in existence for less than 50 years.

8. Strong chemical preservatives are necessary to keep cosmetic products from spoiling.

Cosmetic manufacturers are really counting on you to believe this one. By putting industrial strength synthetic preservatives in their creams and lotions, they can extend their shelf life by several years at a fraction of the cost. The fact is, there are a number of natural alternatives that will keep cosmetic formulas stable. At Aubrey Organics®, our blend of citrus seed extract and vitamins keeps products fresh for a year or more. (And like a few other natural cosmetic manufacturers, we ship direct to stores to gurantee freshness and keep products from sitting around in distributors' warehouses.) The grapefruit seed extract used in the recipes featured here will work just as well. Storing your products in the refrigerator will also keep them from spoiling without the harmful side effects of synthetic preservatives.

9. Synthetic cosmetic products wouldn't be on the market if they weren't safe.

That's what the cosmetic industry would like you to believe. But product safety is a complex issue. Putting some synthetic-laden cream or lotion on your face a few dozen times probably won't give you cancer, or cause your skin to shrivel up or peel off. It's longterm exposure to these chemicals that concerns us—constant, daily absorption for 10, 15, 20 years or more. The fact is that most petrochemicals and other synthetics haven't been around long enough for us to know what effects their extended use can have on our health (or the health of the environment). Another problem is that most cosmetic manufacturers depend on animal testing to determine an ingredient's safety or effectiveness. Testing on animals is not only unethical, it is inaccurate and unreliable. A human's metabolic processes are very different from those of a mouse. Using mice to determine the level at which a chemical is toxic to humans is downright irresponsible. Yet for decades the cosmetic industry has relied exclusively on animal testing to deem their products safe, products whose ingredients' lists can include such chemicals as formaldehyde, mineral oil, coal tar dyes (artificial colors) and hundreds of other synthetics with names so long, they've had to abbreviate them (DEA, TEA) to make them fit on their labels.

10. Dermatologists know how to make or prescribe cosmetics that will keep your skin youthful.

On TV infommercials we often see dermatologists selling some version of the perfect cleanser or moisturizer. A dermatologist is trained to treat skin diseases with drugs, but drugs are not the answer for every skin or scalp condition. Time has shown that many drugs used by medical doctors to treat the skin do not make it youthful or better looking, and sometimes these drugs can have serious side effects and adversely affect the liver, kidneys and other organs. One example of a popular drug used in facial creams and ointments is the much touted Retin-A, an antiwrinkle treatment that leaves the skin extremely sensitive to UV rays and may cause blotchiness and irritation. Topical steroids are another example. Hydrocortisone creams may offer a quick fix to rash-prone or irritated skin, but longterm use can damage your skin's collagen and speed up the aging process. Drugs have their place—they can help reverse damage and even save your life, but they must be used carefully and sparingly. We feel it's best to use drugs to cure or control serious illness, not to put in a face cream to give your skin a lift. Herbals and other natural ingredients are far safer and healthier for you in the long run.

11. Only a professional cosmetic manufacturer can make quality products that really work.

Nothing could be further from the truth. The fact is that a cosmetic product is only as good as the ingredients that go into it. Yet most cosmetic manufacturers are in the business of selling their products at the highest price the market can bear, while keeping their expenses low to generate as large a profit as possible. It's a simple rule of economics—the less you spend in making a product, the higher your profit margin. So cutting corners is the name of the game. Why buy a more expensive natural ingredient when they can use a cheap synthetic in its place? Why preserve cosmetics with citrus seed extract or natural vitamins, which keep them fresh for a year, when they can extend the shelf life of their products by three years or more using a heavy duty chemical preservative with a name longer than your arm? This book will enable you to take charge of your own beauty regimen by showing you how to make your own cosmetics from scratch, quality hair and skin care products with all-natural ingredients that are better for your body than most cosmetics you can buy at your local drug store or department store. In time, your hair and skin will show the difference.

12. People who are allergic to fragrances can't use formulas that contain essential oils.

While some people are allergic to all fragrances, this condition is extremely rare. More than likely, the fragrances they're allergic to are synthetic ones. They are far less likely to be allergic to a natural essential oil than to an artificial fragrance. Almost none of the fragrances found in mass produced cosmetics are natural, which probably explains why many people have allergic reactions to them. One advantage to formulating your own cosmetic products is that you can try different essential oils. If you turn out to be allergic to one, you can replace it with another you can tolerate, or simply opt to not include fragrances in the formula.

13. All you need is a good diet and your skin will be perfect.

A healthy diet and a good nutritional supplementation program (both of which we discuss at length later) are of vital importance to your health, as well as your hair and skin. But proper nutrition is not the only answer. It's a fact that what you put on your hair and skin will directly affect the way you look, and often, the way you feel. Avoiding harsh chemicals and potential carcinogens frequently found in mass produced cosmetics is another important consideration, and one you should take seriously when buying or making your cosmetic products.

14. Lousy skin and dull, thinning hair are inherited traits, and nothing can be done about them.

Though heredity is a factor and you can't completely get around the hair and skin your parents bequeathed upon you, you can do a lot to improve on nature with a sensible hair and skin care regimen and a good diet and exercise discipline.

15. Washing your face in rainwater and brushing your hair 100 times a day are the real secret to beautiful hair and skin.

These great beauty tips have been around since your great-grandmother's time and beyond, but there's much more to good hair and skin. For one thing, rainwater picks up all the chemicals in the atmosphere and often times is not that pure or great. Good water *is* important to the body and the skin, but more important than the type of water you use is WHAT you use to wash your hair and skin. And depending on your hair type, brushing may promote splitting and breakage. (We recommend you massage your scalp instead to help promote hair growth at the root of the problem.) The point is that no one beauty "secret" will work for everybody. You'll simply need to find out what works for you, and that's part of the fun!

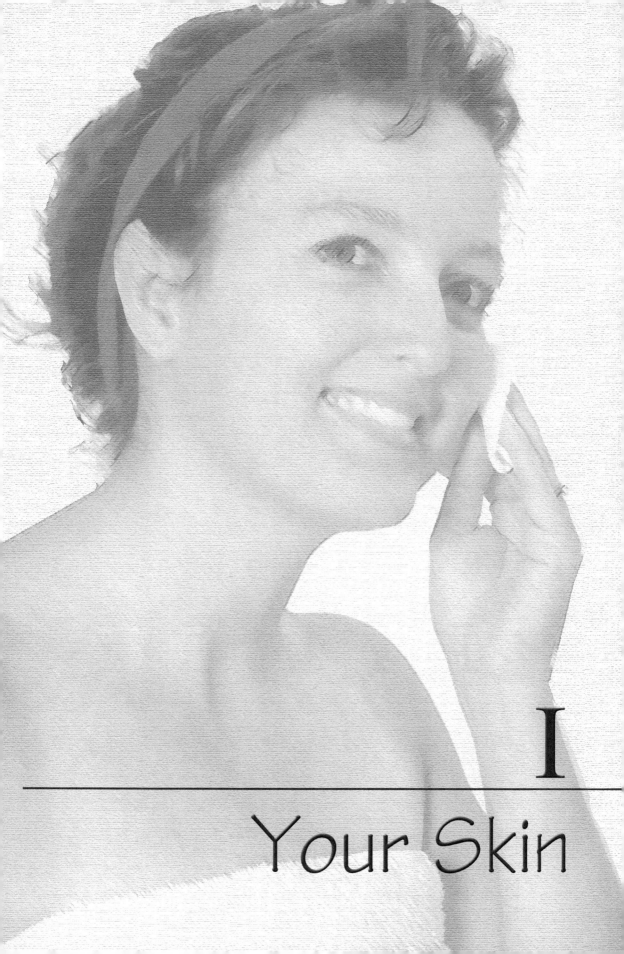

I

Your Skin

"**The deepest aspect of a human being** is the skin," wrote the French poet Paul Valéry. It has been called the body's barrier. Yet, whether you stroke a lover's face or rock a small child in your arms, it is your skin that most profoundly connects you to the world and to others.

The skin is your largest and most important sense organ, the first to develop in the womb and the last you lose in old age. Closely related to your emotional well-being, the life of the skin begins with a parent's loving touch, which prepares you to accept and to give love as an adult. Dozens of studies have determined that babies who are not held and cuddled early on fail to grow and develop at a normal rate, and eventually suffer not only from psychological symptoms, but from physical ones as well, including gastrointestinal and respiratory problems.

More Than Skin Deep

The skin also acts as a kind of litmus paper for your general health. If you're allergic to something, often you'll break out in a rash. If you don't feel well, your skin may turn pale or look dull and pasty. The state of your skin reveals your state of health, and all sorts of instant decisions are made about you based on your complexion.

Your face is your fortune—it influences how people feel about you and how you feel about yourself. Even babies don't escape judgment: it has long been known that a cute child can misbehave more than one that isn't. Studies have shown that attractive people are hired first. Thus, your face can open the door to a great job, or cause you to be the person remembered across a crowded room.

Skin problems can derail your self-esteem, sometimes permanently. Teenagers with acne suffer psychologically, sometimes to the point of suicide, due to the appearance of their skin. Men and women with wrinkled skin or thinning hair can develop low self-esteem, and will pay almost anything to turn these conditions around.

This vulnerability to vanity is well-known by the cosmetic industry. Women are constantly bombarded with ads that picture youthful, anorexic models next to a jar of some dream cream and a few lines of impressive-sounding copy. Men endure less of this sort of advertising, yet ads for men's hair care products rarely fail to show a hunky guy with a very full head of hair.

What's annoying about these ads is that their primary purpose is to promote anxiety in the readers about their appearance, because no one truly measures up. Not even supermodels look picture-perfect all the time. That takes an incredible amount of effort and more than a little airbrushing, and then the effect is good for only a few short years. Obviously, the ads promise what the products can't deliver. Another disturbing aspect is that, almost without exception, the ads rarely focus on what's really in the products. The text consists of a few well-chosen buzz words that tout the flavor-of-the-month magic ingredient.

Let's face it (pun intended). We know practically nothing about the products that we put on our bodies, despite the fact that how we look to others and to ourselves is incredibly important to us. Couple this ignorance with the lack of understanding we have about our skin and how it functions, and we have an appalling state of affairs. Warning: the next few pages are a little technical, but put on your thinking caps and make an effort to get to know that masterpiece of complex bioengineering: your skin.

Under Your Skin

The skin is a complex organ that performs a dazzling array of functions, many seemingly contradictory. While it is itself an organ, it also holds the other organs together and protects them from the external elements. Often called the "second kidney," the skin is the second most important organ of elimination through its release of perspiration—yet it is quite water-resistant.

An organ with so much to do is anything but simple. Within a single square inch of skin are approximately 19 million cells, including 650 sweat glands, 100 sebum or oil glands, 65 hair follicles, 19,000 sensory cells and as much as 13 feet of microscopic blood vessels. Here are some more skin facts:

- The skin of an adult weighs around eight pounds and would measure 20 square feet if stretched out.
- Over an average lifetime, approximately 40 pounds of skin cells are shed.
- The thickness of the skin measures from 1/25th of an inch (the eyelids) to 1/8th of an inch (the soles of the feet).
- The skin also functions as a nutritional factory, producing vitamin D-3, a necessary ingredient in the formation of bone, and has an active role in the metabolism of carbohydrates and amino acids.

The skin is made up of two layers: the epidermis and the dermis. Each layer has its own set of vital functions, but one easy way to remember the difference is that the epidermis has nerve endings but no blood vessels, while the dermis has both. The outermost layer of the epidermis, called the stratum corneum, is made up of numerous sheets of interwoven keratin—the same protein that's found in the hair and nails. This layer is what makes the skin tough and waterproof, and its function is so important that 95% of the skin cells are involved in producing it.

Here's the life cycle of a keratin cell: it is born in the deepest part of the epidermis (beneath the stratum corneum). For the first two weeks of its life, it migrates upwards. The last two weeks of its life are spent on the surface of the skin, becoming increasingly flattened out, dying, then ultimately being shed. The stratum corneum is constantly shedding cells—between two and three billion cells or cellular fragments daily. While the outermost surface of the skin is dead, it is kept moist by a thin layer of sebum (oil) and perspiration, which is transported from deeper layers in the dermis and secreted by the pores. Sometimes the stratum corneum can look dull and drab due to the accumulation of dead skin cells. A program of cleansing, steaming, masking and moisturizing the skin will encourage proper shedding.

Within the epidermis are also the melanocytes, cells that produce pigment, which are more active in people with darker skin, but not more numerous. During sun exposure, the melanocytes inject the pigment, known as melanin, into the skin's keratin cells to protect them from further damage. The tan they produce in lighter-skinned people is nothing but an indication that the epidermis has been somewhat damaged by sunlight. You've heard it before, and you'll hear it again in this book: there is no such thing as a healthy tan.

Also found in the epidermis, the Langerhans cells are part of the skin's active immune system. These cells are shaped like tiny octopi, complete with tentacles that reach around their keratin cell neighbors. When a bit of foreign matter is absorbed into the epidermis, it sticks to the tentacles of these cells and is carried to other parts of the body via the lymphatic system, where it is neutralized by white blood cells. So while your skin's active immune system is able to identify and eliminate toxins, an overload of pollutants—including chemicalized cosmetic products—can hinder its ability to do the job.

Just beneath the epidermis, the dermis is where the glands do their work. The sebaceous glands, or oil glands, are in charge of manufacturing sebum, the body's own natural moisturizing factor. The purpose of sebum is to prevent evaporation of the water in the skin, and also to protect the body from absorbing excess moisture. The raw materials necessary for the synthesis of sebum are amino acids, essential fatty acids and carbohydrates. Too dry or too greasy skin is often the result of imbalanced fat consumption, and we'll discuss the importance of this in a later chapter. The dermis is also where the sweat glands produce perspiration, which seeps to the surface of the skin through the pores to help maintain a constant temperature in the body, and to help keep the skin moisturized.

The dermis is comprised primarily of three kinds of protein—collagen, elastin and reticulin. Reticulin fibers hold together bundles of collagen, while elastin, as its name suggests, gives elasticity to the dermis. Collagen is the most prevalent dermal protein, making up around 70% of the dermis. Cross-linking, or degeneration, of collagen is what creates wrinkles in the skin.

What causes the dermis to deteriorate? Too much sun, to start. Sun is the natural enemy of young collagen because it causes oxidation of the fat particles in your skin, which in turn leads to free radical (electron) damage to the skin's collagen. Another cause of free radical damage to the skin is the toxins absorbed from the polluted world in which we live. The use of synthetic cosmetic products only makes a bad situation worse.

What is the price of progress? If we look at an old photograph of an upper-class 19th century woman, chances are, even late in her life, her skin would be smoother and more wrinkle-free than that of her free-wheeling, 20th century sister. What's to blame? Sun and cosmetics. Well-brought-up 19th century women shunned the sun, and the skin care products available 100 or more years ago were natural, since that was all that was available.

What's important to remember about the skin is that it is a living part of your body with several interrelated circulating systems (blood, sweat, sebum, nerve and lymph), any of which can be damaged by absorption of chemicals, or enhanced by a good skin care system. The question of absorption into the skin, however, is a tricky one. Up until recently, the medical industry had largely denied it even happens!

The Modern Question

Traditional cultures around the world never questioned whether or not substances applied to the skin were absorbed into the body. They knew: whole systems of medicine were organized around effective methods of applying herbal medicines directly to the skin. Thousands of years ago the Chinese were increasing the benefits of acupuncture with moxibustion, the process of applying burning herbs to particular points on the skin, and Native American tribes applied heated herbal poultices to injured areas to increase circulation and absorption.

Yet modern Western medicine has considered the skin impervious to absorption, even as recently as 1957, when Dr. Stephen Rothman, keynote speaker at the 11th International Congress of Dermatology, held in Sweden, asserted that nothing from the outside could penetrate through the skin. Forty years later, absorption is so much taken for granted that today many drugs are administered via skin patches, including nicotine (in antismoking treatments), estrogen and nitroglycerin.

Unfortunately, much of the current understanding of the skin's permeability (its ability to absorb substances) is due to the damage powerful pesticides and other man-made chemicals have inflicted on exposed workers. One of the best publicized examples involved 40 men in a chemical plant in Occidental, California, in 1960. This plant produced dibromochloropropane (DBCP), a powerful but dangerous pesticide. The men exposed to DBCP had been unable to father children, and while airborne levels of the chemical had been kept beneath occupational limits, the danger from skin exposure was ignored, with tragic consequences.

Another chemical, hexachlorophene, an antibacterial used in soaps throughout the 1950s and 60s, was shown to cause brain damage—and even death—in babies through absorption into the skin. Malathion, an organophosphate insecticide routinely sprayed for years in California and Florida over millions of acres to control Medfly infestation, is also absorbed through the skin, and has been linked to many serious health problems, including upper respiratory disorders and memory loss.

Herbicides, wood preservatives, pesticides, disinfectants and solvents are among many chemicals known to be assimilated into the body through exposure by the skin. What many of these chemicals have in common is a strong ability to dissolve lipids, or fats. This characteristic is what enables them to penetrate the skin. The skin, as you read earlier, is interpenetrated with tiny channels that conduct sweat and sebum from deep within to its surface. The sides of these channels are lined with water or fat molecules, and those substances capable of dissolving in either of these two mediums may also be absorbed into the skin.

Increased awareness of illnesses caused by skin exposure to dangerous chemicals is important, and various governmental agencies are to be commended for their attention to the safety of workers. However, absorption into the skin of chemicals used in everyday hair and skin care products has been insufficiently studied. As we mentioned earlier, there are around 75,000 chemicals that we might come in contact with on a given day, and their effects on the body are unknown. Even very, very low-level exposure to a variety of these chemicals can cause a number of health problems, both immediate and long term. No one knows for certain, and anyone who says otherwise does not fully understand the effects of skin absorption on the body.

One reason you don't hear much about this hazard may lie in the accepted definition of cosmetics by the Food and Drug Administration. According to the FDA, cosmetics are, "Articles which are intended to be rubbed, poured, sprinkled or sprayed or introduced to, or otherwise applied to, the human body for cleaning, beautifying, promoting attractiveness or altering the appearance *without affecting the body's structure or function"* (our italics). This definition is over 60 years old, the result of the old thinking about the skin that dominated medicine until very recently. Now this thinking has become entrenched in bureaucracy, and while a few changes have been made for a few workers on a case-by-case basis, little has been done to protect consumers from the chemicals common in our marketplace. The cosmetics industry has simply gotten too big and too powerful.

Reading Between the Lines

The cosmetics game is not about making consumers healthier or more beautiful; it's primarily a word game. Here's how it works: Advertise the product with language that hints it will do miracles, but get ready to withdraw the advertisement if the FDA rules that a drug claim has been made.

According to the official definition of a cosmetic, if a product claims to alter the body's structure or function, then its classification will be changed to that of a drug, a pronouncement no cosmetic manufacturer wants to hear, because this would subject their products to a much more stringent and expensive set of regulations. This current definition certainly limits advertising claims, but it also provides cosmetic manufacturers with an out: cosmetic products are safe because they aren't absorbed into the skin because they're cosmetics—a meaningless, circular, Catch-22 argument.

More cosmetic products are made in the U.S. than anywhere in the world. As a result, American cosmetic manufacturers are protected by a very strong trade organization, the Cosmetic, Toiletry and Fragrance Association (CTFA), whose main function is to ensure governmental acceptance of as wide a variety of ingredients as possible for the formulating freedom of its members. (This organization advocates testing on animals.)

A brief look at different editions of their *CTFA Dictionary* shows the CTFA's primary orientation is towards synthetic chemicals. In 1977, when the Cosmetic Labeling Act became law and manufacturers were forced to list ingredients, the dictionary mostly listed synthetic chemicals. Very few herbs made the dictionary that year. In the 20 years since, however, the dictionary has tripled in size, and many of the new listings are herbal ingredients.

We don't want to knock the CTFA; that's not our purpose here. We just want you to think about the implications of a trade organization with a strong influence on the federal government, an organization dominated by the old-fashioned notion that the skin is like an old shoe that can be polished with any old thing because, after all, nothing can be absorbed.

So far we've talked about the bad news: that cosmetics are full of synthetic ingredients, and that the degree to which these chemicals can be absorbed into your skin is relatively unstudied. However, the good news is that herbs, many of which are highly beneficial for your skin, can be absorbed as well. Apply just a drop of an essential oil to your skin, and it can be detected in another part of your body almost immediately. That's why herbs are such valuable ingredients in natural cosmetics: they work, and usually more gently and with fewer side effects than synthetic chemicals.

Check out the label of most commercial cosmetics and you'll find a long list of man-made ingredients, most of which have been around for 25 years or less. That's a nanosecond in the evolution of this planet, and perhaps one second in our own human evolution. Whether or not we have developed the appropriate immune response and have biologically learned to adapt to these synthetic substances is simply not known. It just makes sense that the products you put on your skin should be made of ingredients that have been around at least as long as you have.

Yet manufacturers of mass produced cosmetics won't use exclusively natural materials—they're too expensive. Also, all-natural formulas are too unstable to withstand the long shelf lives needed for mass distribution of these products, which sometimes sit around in warehouses for two or three years before they even make it into stores. Most synthetic chemicals are used in cosmetics either because they're cheaper or because they make some phase of mass manufacturing or distribution possible. For example, strong synthetic preservatives were developed to extend shelf life, while synthetic emulsifiers such as stearalkonium chloride were created to keep the mixtures of oil and water in creams and lotions from separating.

Foam builders, thickeners, opacifiers, sequestering agents, synthetic colors: these are among the many functions of chemicals commonly used in mass produced cosmetics. They do nothing for the health of your hair and skin, but are there simply to make products look good enough to sell. Our argument is that, given the overall contamination of the environment with man-made chemicals, you're better off without them. Remember: what you don't know *can* hurt you. That's why it's important to use natural products on your hair and skin. And you can't buy products more natural than those you make yourself.

How Skin Ages

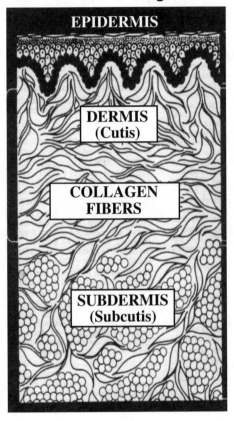

EPIDERMIS

DERMIS
(Cutis)

COLLAGEN
FIBERS

SUBDERMIS
(Subcutis)

In the diagram at the left you can see the three layers of the skin: epidermis, dermis, and subdermis. Just below the dermis are the collagen fibers, which contain the three important dermal proteins, *collagen, reticulin* and *elastin.*

Collagen is very important to the youthful look of your skin. As long as the collagen fibers are non-cross-linked, the skin will remain healthy and supple, with almost no wrinkles, and the "spring back" elasticity of youthful skin. However, if the collagen fibers become cross-linked, non-flexible, dull, wrinkled skin will result. One element that causes collagen to become cross-linked is UV ray exposure, therefore it is advisable to avoid excessive sun exposure and to use a sunblock with an SPF (sun protection factor) of 15 or more when going outdoors.

Another factor that can damage your "soluble collagen" and cause it to become cross-linked is exposure to chemicals, particularly the various synthetic chemicals in cosmetics that can be absorbed into the skin. Absorption can affect your skin's collagen in a positive way or a negative way. When you use natural cosmetics you are actually protecting your skin's collagen in two ways: by keeping it from exposure to harmful chemicals, and by providing the many benefits herbs, vitamins and other natural ingredients can have on your skin.

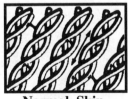

**Normal Skin
(Non-Cross-Linked
Collagen)**

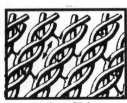

**Aging Skin
(Cross-Linked
Collagen)**

25

Diagram of the Skin

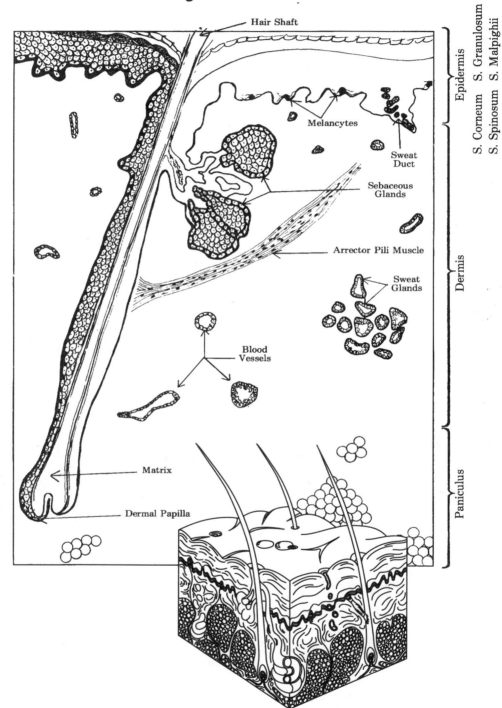

Hair Shaft

Epidermis

S. Corneum   S. Granulosum
S. Spinosum   S. Malpighii

Melancytes

Sweat
Duct

Sebaceous
Glands

Arrector Pili Muscle

Dermis

Sweat
Glands

Blood
Vessels

Matrix

Paniculus

Dermal Papilla

Cross-Section of the Skin

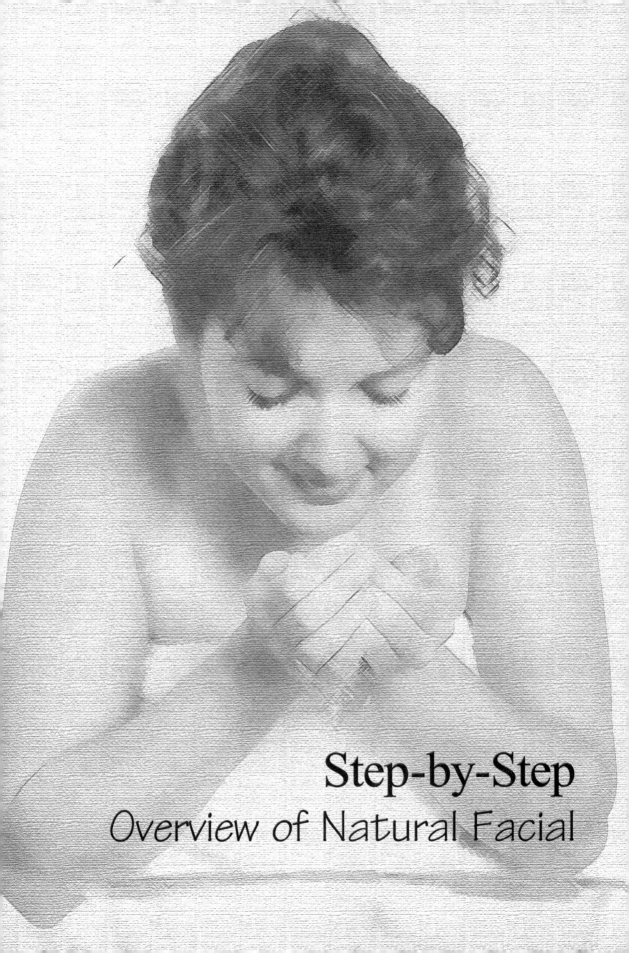

Step-by-Step
Overview of Natural Facial

The Natural Facial

Nothing will give you faster results than this natural facial, Aubrey's step-by-step skin care method using all natural formulas. This complete beauty regimen gives your skin a complete workout—from steaming, cleansing and exfoliating to toning and moisturizing. Follow this natural method daily using the formulas you've created for your particular skin type, and you'll be amazed with the way your skin looks and feels.

Step 1— Steam

Steaming your skin is the first step, and it's an important one. It relaxes the tissues, helps detoxify the complexion and opens pores to prepare skin for cleansing. For best results, use Aubrey's Facial Flowers Steam Concentrate (Formula #14) when steaming your complexion.

After removing makeup (we recommend you use jojoba oil for this purpose), carefully pour a capful or two of Facial Flowers Steam Concentrate into a bowl of very hot water, then place a towel over your head, creating a tent. Close your eyes and allow the steam to flow over your face for 10 minutes or so.

If you are pressed for time, a quick facial steaming can also be done with a hot towel. Just soak a clean towel in very hot water, wring it out until it's damp dry, then place it on your face for 1 to 2 minutes.

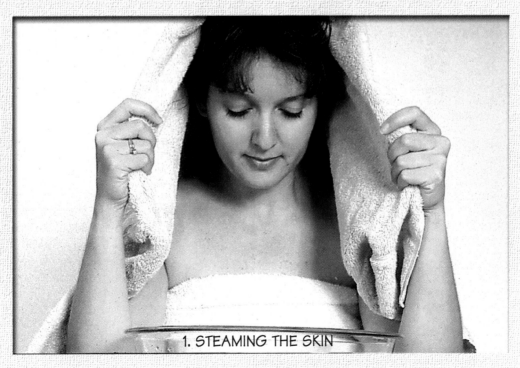

1. STEAMING THE SKIN

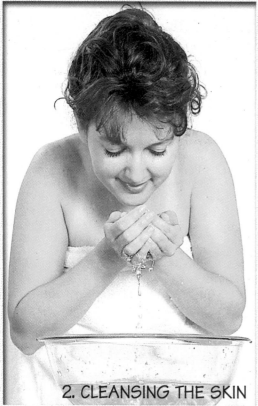

2. CLEANSING THE SKIN

Step 2- Cleanse

Bar soaps can be drying to the skin, so when cleansing your complexion, it's best to use a mild facial cleanser instead. In the Formulas section we offer two different recipes, for normal to oily and normal to dry skin respectively.

After steaming, apply a small amount of cleanser to fingers or washcloth and work across face and neck, massaging gently into skin. Rinse thoroughly in warm water.

Once of twice a week, you'll want to use an herbal mask to help clear the pores, break up oil deposits and help remove dead skin cells that can make your complexion look dull and lifeless. This is a good time to exfoliate and deep-cleanse the skin.

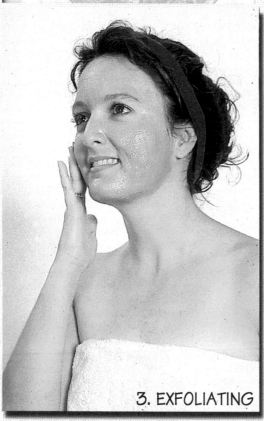

3. EXFOLIATING

Step 3— Exfoliate
(Once or twice a week)

The best and most gentle way to exfoliate the skin is to use either a facial mask or gentle scrub (some of our masks double as both). In our Formulas section we offer four different recipes according to your skin type. Here Priscilla is using Green Clay & Blue Green Algae Moisturizing Mask (Formula #7), a deep-cleansing mask for all skin types, applying a thin layer throughout face and neck with her fingers. Once the mask is in place, you may leave it on for about 15 minutes, then wipe it off with a damp cloth and rinse skin thoroughly.

Step 4— Tone

Toners are among the worst culprits in the cosmetic industry, known to use synthetic alcohols and other harsh chemicals. But a good herbal toner will wipe away excess oils and debris, remove soap residues and clear and purify the complexion. It is an important step that is often overlooked, even during professional facials. Be sure to choose a toner that's right for your skin type. Then dampen a cotton ball or pad with toner and wipe across face and neck in upward strokes, changing cotton as it becomes soiled.

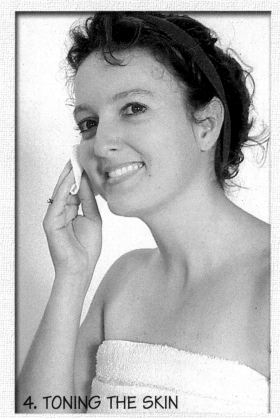

4. TONING THE SKIN

Step 5— Moisturize

Moisturizing is an important step because it actually nourishes your skin and restores its right moisture balance. Apply a small amount of moisturizer to fingertips and work it gently into face and neck, massaging skin lightly. Priscilla is using Janine's Night & Day Cream SPF 15 (Formula #12), a hardworking formula that doubles as a daytime moisturizer and night cream.

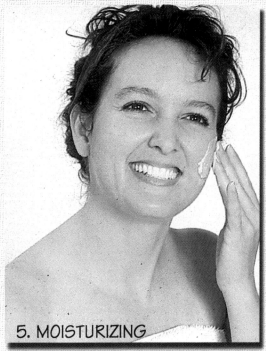

Step 6— Hydrate

After applying your moisturizer, we recommend a spritz with a good hydrating spray. Aubrey's Sparkling Mineral Water Herbal Facial Spray (Formula #13) gives your skin added moisture and helps your moisturizer do its job more effectively.

5. MOISTURIZING

31

The Natural Facial Massage

The following diagrams will show you step-by-step how to give yourself a professional facial massage. For optimum benefit, we recommend you do the massage as part of your facial, after cleansing your skin but before applying the mask and/or toner. Practice the movements and don't worry if at first you don't seem very good at it—your technique will improve in time. If you have dry skin, massage with a nourishing oil, such as jojoba oil, and if your skin isn't so dry, try a light massage cream. If you paid for a professional facial, it's very likely the aesthetician would include a massage as part of your treatment. But she or he would most likely be using some chemical-laden cream or massage oil on your face. This is the best massage in the business at any price, and the only one that can guarantee all natural products that won't harm delicate facial skin.

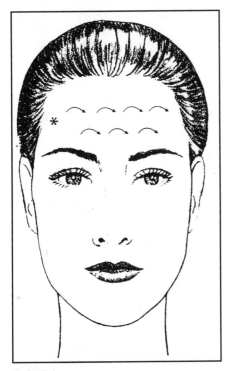

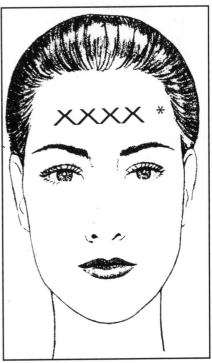

STEP 1
Circular massage of the forehead

STEP 2
Crisscross massage of the forehead

Using the middle and index fingers of both hands in a semicircular movement, apply light strokes (effleurage) to the skin across the forehead. Begin at the right temple, moving left, to finish at the left temple. Do this across the forehead five times. Do not lift your fingers: movement must be smooth and even.

Using the index and middle fingers of both hands, begin at the left temple and work from left to right using crisscross motions and pressing lightly. Do this five times. Do not lift your fingers: movement must be smooth and even.

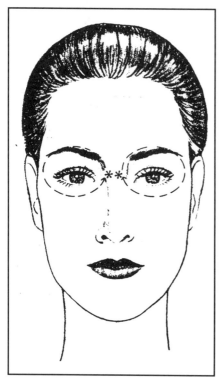

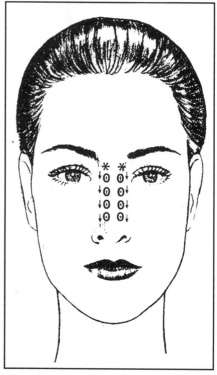

STEP 3
Eye area massage

Using a very light touch on the thin, delicate skin around the eyes, place middle fingers at each inner corner of the eyes and index fingers over the brows. Then slide fingers gently to the outer corner of the eyes and back again. Do this five times.

STEP 4
Massage of nose area

Place your index and middle fingers on each side of the bridge of the nose. Press firmly and rotate one time, then slide a quarter inch down the nose with a light, circular movement (effleurage). Press and rotate once, slide down, and repeat. End by pressing and rotating on the tip of your nose, then return to the beginning position, and repeat three times.

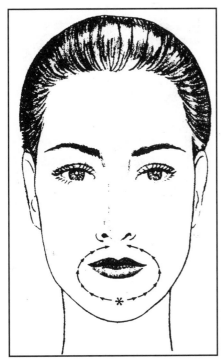

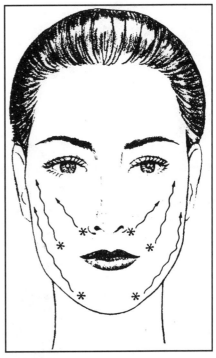

STEP 5
Massage around mouth area

Slide your right hand under your chin, and bring thumb and middle fingers up to the corners of your mouth. Do a light, circular movement (effleurage) five times. Continue around the mouth, pressing and rotating until you reach the cleft in your upper lip. Repeat three times.

STEP 6
Massage the cheeks

Using the middle and index fingers of both hands, massage from the chin across the cheeks to the earlobes, from the corners of the mouth to the earlobes, and from the corners of the nose to the tips of the ears. Repeat five times.

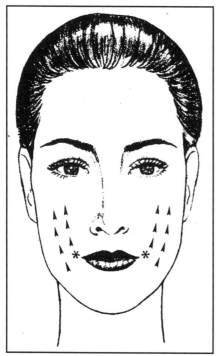

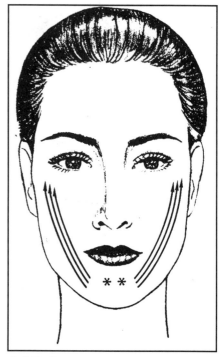

STEP 7
Stimulating massage of the cheeks

Beginning at the corners of the mouth, gently but firmly tap the sides of the face with a lifting and dropping motion of the hands. Do both sides simultaneously. Repeat five times.

STEP 8
Massage the sides of the face

Grasp the flesh at the chin with thumb and the knuckle of the first finger of both hands. Work up the face with a "plucking" movement. Go up both sides of the face in this manner, then come down, repeating the movement five times.

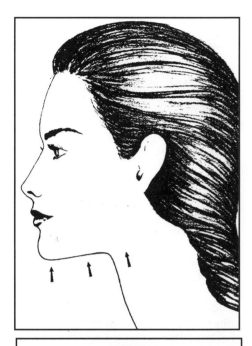

STEP 9— **Massage under jaw line**

Gently lift the jaw line with the tips of the fingers and slide back toward the ears. Repeat five times.

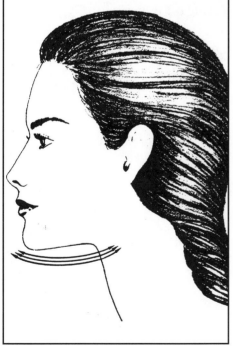

STEP 10 — **Massage under jaw**

Place both hands (palms down) with the fingertips intertwined under the neck. Begin a scissors-like movement back and forth, keeping the fingertips together. Repeat this movement five times.

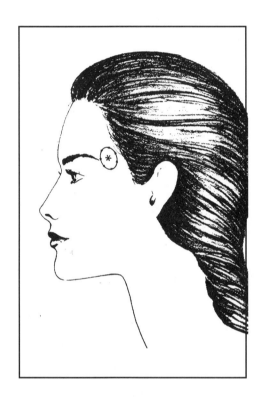

STEP 11— **Completing facial massage**

Finish off your facial massage by gently rotating temples, then pressing for three seconds. Repeat five times, gradually tapering off pressure.

Acupuncture and Your Skin

I carry a package of acupuncture needles with me along with a tiny cocktail straw to act as the "blow-gun" for tapping them into my skin. Using this ancient Chinese science, I have learned how to erase a headache and relieve a stiff neck, backache, or even a toothache by tapping the needles into certain points in the body. Does this sound dangerous? Some people carry bottles of aspirin or Xanax around. If you think about it, the tapping of a tiny needle about the width of a horse-hair into your body is far safer than most of the drugs people toss down their throats. Choosing pills over needles is our cultural bias. Nevertheless, I must now introduce my disclaimer: If you want to try acupuncture, go to a qualified physician with a knowledge of this ancient science. In other words, don't do as I do: do as I suggest.

Western physicians still do little work with acupuncture, and one reason for this is that acupuncture is not 100% explainable. Eastern medicine does not, like Western medicine, feel the need to explain. The need to know *why* something helps the sick, *why* certain herbs work, and the need to prove through testing (first on animals) the *why* and *how* of any substance or technique is not part of the Eastern philosophy. It is peculiarly Western and most apparent in the United States to test everything. We disapprove or approve based on these tests, many of which are highly inaccurate (again, think animal testing and the process of determining whether a drug is safe on humans because it works on a rat). Still, we arrive at certain conclusions we hold as fact based on these tests, and make medical decisions accordingly.

Eastern medicine, practiced widely and successfully for thousands of years, often puts little importance on our so-called "scientific" tests. The Chinese, who think in terms of processes rather than in terms of substances, could never accept our concept of testing and statistics. If a Western physician is going to accept and use acupuncture, he or she is going to be put in the position of accepting a whole different way of looking at the body without knowing, in the Western way, why.

Yin and yang, the complementary opposites on which Chinese medicine is based, are one essential difference between East and West. Medically speaking, there are five yin organs: heart, lungs, spleen, liver and kidneys. These organs store but do not transmit. There are six yang organs (which transform but do not retain): gall bladder, stomach, small intestine, large intestine, bladder and Triple Warmer. The Western physician must also accept the five fundamental substances: chi, blood, jing, shen and a group of substances not specifically named but which represent a variety of elements, e.g., saliva and perspiration. He or she must also accept the five phases (sometimes wrongly translated as five elements): wood, fire, earth, metal and water.

Phases, changes and processes provide an entirely different understanding of what we call substances and elements. Wood (such as that of a tree) is associated with growth; fire is the peak of activity (including incipient decline); metal is associated with decline; water with rest and incipient growth; and earth, which links all the others together, is both a beginning and an end. Chinese herbal medicine, which is accepted even less than acupuncture by Western doctors, is also based on yin and yang and the temporal cycles.

Acupuncture works whether or not you understand the philosophy of Chinese medicine and yin and yang, and many Western nations are now involved in the art of the needles. So why isn't more acupuncture practiced in the U.S.? Mark Duke (author of *Acupuncture: The Chinese Art of Healing*) asked the news editor of the American Medical Association (AMA) weekly newsletter some years ago why more acupuncture isn't used by physicians, since it obviously works and has since 1600 B. C. The AMA answered:

"We don't understand it and we don't know anything about it. We know that it exists and that it has for a long time. But it has not come up so far in this part of the world. Acupuncture ranks with Oriental folklore, but it can't be called medicine. There is a very heavy psychological element in it, possibly involving self-hypnosis. Is there any real scientific basis for it? It doesn't really matter. You know, if it helps you with the discomforts of an ailment, you don't really care whether it's scientific or not."

Here's another theory as to why acupuncture is not accepted by the medical industry. If this art were to become widely practiced in the United States, the average doctor's income would fall. Surgeons and anesthesiologists would be drastically affected, since in China and other Eastern countries, acupuncture is sometimes used in place of general anesthesia, and in many cases, can prevent surgery altogether. With the use of acupuncture, the 15,000,000 pounds of aspirin sold every year would drop tremendously, as would the sale of most pain relievers. The nearly two billion prescriptions (and half-a-billion refills) issued by doctors would be greatly diminished. Life-sign monitoring devices, which make up 20% of the cost of an operation, in many cases would no longer be needed. Hospital stays would be reduced by up to 30% due to the elimination of chemical anesthetics.

Still, the United States is one of the few countries that refuses to study acupuncture or offer research grants to understand it better. However, an individual wishing to try this highly effective and noninvasive method of treatment should be able to find a good acupuncture practitioner even though conventional medicine does not recognize it.

The Acupressure Face Lift

Even if you are familiar with the principles of acupuncture discussed here, you may not be aware that, in addition to improving your overall health, acupuncture can be used to tone your facial muscles, help reduce premature lines and wrinkles and keep your complexion clear and younger looking. The good news (for the squeamish few) is that you don't actually need dozens of needles sticking out of your face, arms, legs and back to get the full benefits of this ancient art.

Acupressure is another art that works, and one that you can do yourself as part of your health and beauty regimen. Using the same basic principles of acupuncture, the Acupressure Face Lift works by stimulating the meridian points on your face and other parts of the body that are considered "skin care points" in acupuncture treatments. Applying pressure with a blunt, pointed object—anything from a makeup brush handle to your knuckle or thumb—will take the place of needles. (There is now on the market a "spark" tool which can be used to stimulate the acupressure points. For your money, the method of pressing with a blunt object works just as well.)

To do your face lift, simply apply moderate pressure to the specific meridian point for about ten seconds, using a clockwise circular motion as you press. Move from left to right, stimulating the points opposite each other as shown in the diagrams. (For example, start at point 1 on the left side of your forehead, and then go to point 2 on the right side of the forehead, etc.)

Today many aestheticians use acupressure during facial massage. It is a simple and effective treatment you can add to your regular skin care regimen which, in some ways, is even more effective than facial exercises. The best time to do the Acupressure Face Lift is after you've done your facial, but never after you've eaten or when you're tired. Put aside some time at the beginning of your day or early in the evening and do it daily for best results.

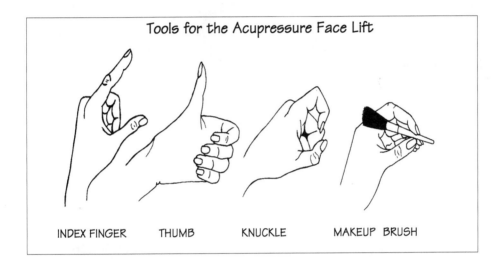

Tools for the Acupressure Face Lift

INDEX FINGER   THUMB   KNUCKLE   MAKEUP BRUSH

On the next page you'll find a front and side view of the location of the Acupressure Face Lift points. There are approximately 29 points on the front of your face and neck. When you stimulate these points, the face muscles relax, and the flow of lipids increases, which is very important to proper skin respiration.

In the next few diagrams we will show you how to work these acupressure points, starting from the forehead and moving down to the neck. The points around the eyes (five around each eye) will help reduce wrinkles and dark circles. The four points near the lips will help you smooth those fine lines that form around the mouth.

41

The Acupressure Face Lift Points

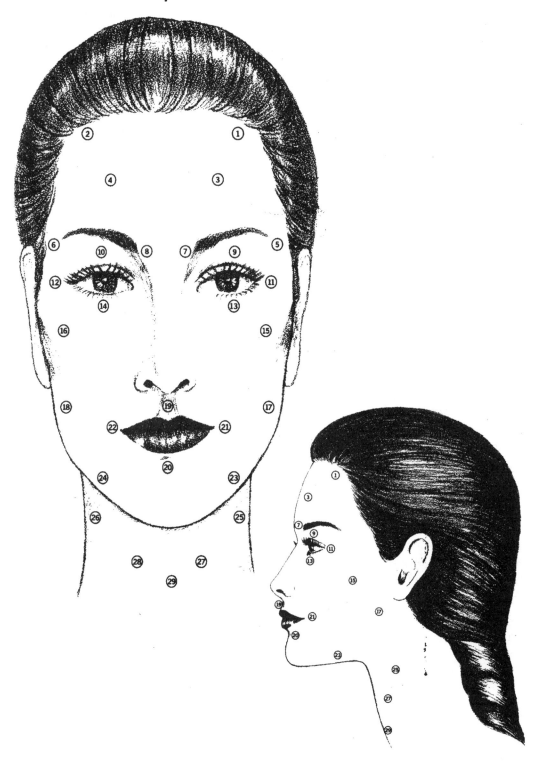

42

1. The Forehead Area

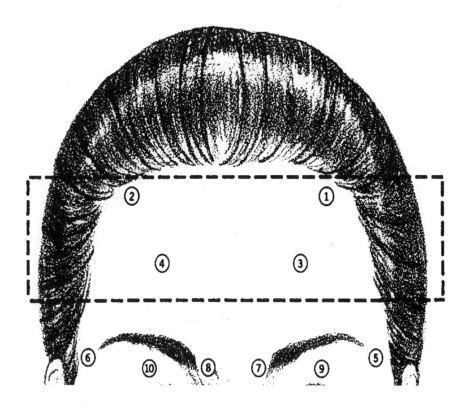

You should begin your Acupressure Face Lift at the forehead, then progress across and downward. We will discuss the specific treatment points and what they represent in acupuncture, although here we are primarily using them as a dermatological/beauty treatment. We will refer to the points by number. (Remember these numbers are for our use here, and do not refer to other numbers that might appear on other acupuncture charts.)

Points 1 and 2 are not only stimulating to the skin and help soften lines along the forehead, but are similar to classic acupuncture points on the back of the neck, in the webbing between the thumb and forefinger, and on the spine (atop the third lumbar vertebra, often used to relieve headaches, migraines and other types of pain). Move on to points 3 and 4. These serve the same function as 1 and 2 and complement them. As you move through these four points, stimulate each one for about ten seconds.

2. The Eye Area

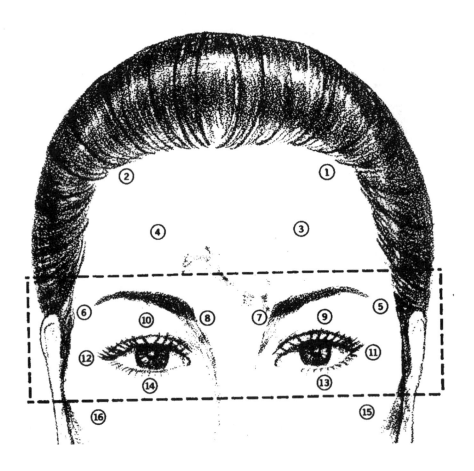

Starting at point 5 on the outer edge of the left eyebrow, stimulate this point, then move to point 6 on the outer edge of the right eyebrow. Continue on to point 7 on the inner edge of the left eyebrow, and then move the short distance to point 8 on the inner edge of the right eyebrow. Points 9 and 10 are just below the eyebrow, close to the center of the eye, just beyond the notch that can be felt in the skull opening. Stimulate these areas more gently and with great care, as the skin there is more delicate. The points in the eye area will help reduce lines around the eyes. Points 9 and 10 are also indicated for treatment of allergy, sinusitis, the neck and the lower back. Move on to points 11 and 12, then points 13 and 14.

3. The Mouth Area

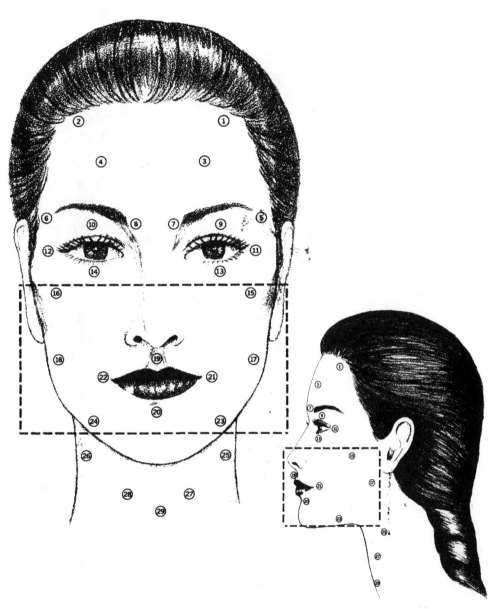

Move on to point 15, which is on the high part of the cheekbone area, in line with the center of the ear, then continue on to point 16. Proceed to point 17, which is slightly below the ear, then point 18 on the other side. Point 19 is midway between the nose and upper lip, and point 20 can be found just below it. Point 20 is also the sneeze control center, so if you have a fit of sneezing, stimulating this point will help. Move on to points 21 and 22, on either side of the mouth, then to 23 and 24, on the edge of the jaw line.

4. The Neck Area

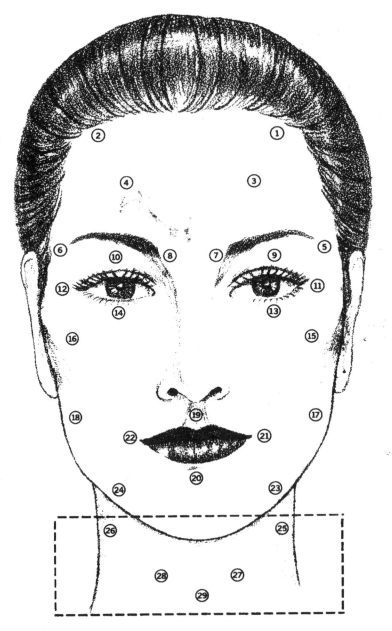

Next, go to point 25 on the left side of the neck, and to point 26 on the right side of the neck. Then proceed to the front of the neck to points 27 and 28, and finish with point 29. This completes your Acupressure Face Lift. We strongly suggest you try this ancient facial treatment once or twice a week. It will do wonders for your complexion!

Other Important Points

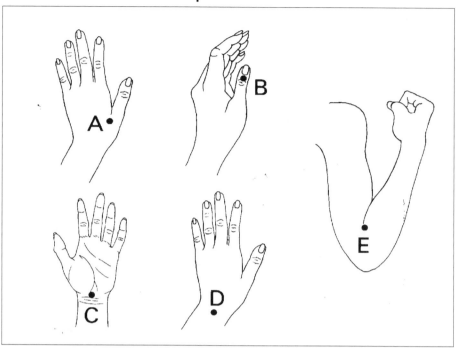

There are quite a few more points that, while located on other parts of the body, have quite a bit to do with the skin. Stimulating these other points will complete the perfect skin care treatment. In the diagram above we have lettered them, beginning with A to avoid confusion with the facial points we discussed previously.

In the webbing between the thumb and forefinger of both hands you will find point A, one of the most important points in acupuncture and acupressure. This is the first place that should be stimulated to help relieve headache pain. It is a sedation point which relaxes the entire body. Between the nail and the first joint of the thumb, just behind the nail on the side farthest from the other fingers, is a very delicate spot we will call point B. Again, this point is often used to get rid of a headache.

On the most prominent crease of the inner wrist, directly in line with the middle finger, is point C. This is an important point for the skin, and in acupuncture and G-Jo (the Chinese word for first aid), it is one of several points stimulated to help treat eczema. Point D is on the back of the arm, about two thumb widths above the most prominent crease of the upper wrist, and in line with the middle finger. This is another important skin care area. Point E is on the extreme end of the outer crease of the elbow. This point, along with point A, is used in the treatment of acne.

Point F is on the back center of the neck, where the spine joins the skull (cervical atlas). Put your hand back there now and locate it. Press on this point, rotating your finger slightly as you press. Now remove fingers and rotate your head. Notice how relaxed your neck feels? If you combine the "F spot" with A, D and G, you can quickly treat a stiff neck or a headache. Point G is a very delicate point and should never be used on a child. If you put your finger there, press firmly, rotate, then release it, you will notice your neck becoming as relaxed as when you pressed point F.

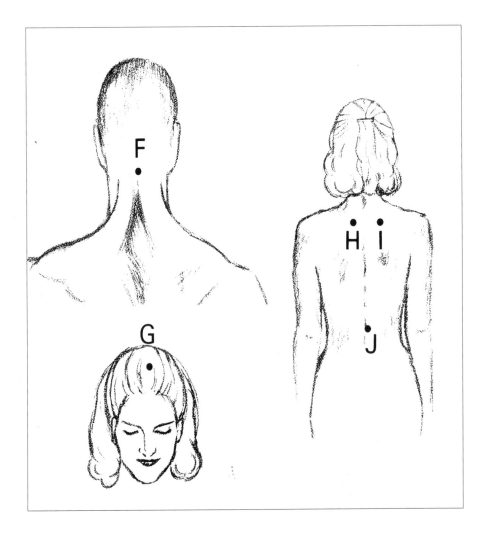

Point K can be found on the center of the crease at the rear of the knee. This is a stimulation point for skin problems, and it also helps with the relief of low back pain and tension. However, this point should not be used if you have varicose veins. Point L is another skin care point, located in the hollow behind the crown of the outer ankle, and is also a general pain control center.

Point M is located in the inner thigh, about the width of two thumbs above the top of the kneecap, in line with the crown of the inner ankle. This skin treatment point has been used to treat acne.

As you use and become acquainted with these various treatment points, finding them will become second nature. But for the time being, refer to these diagrams when doing your acupressure treatments. You'll be amazed with the results.

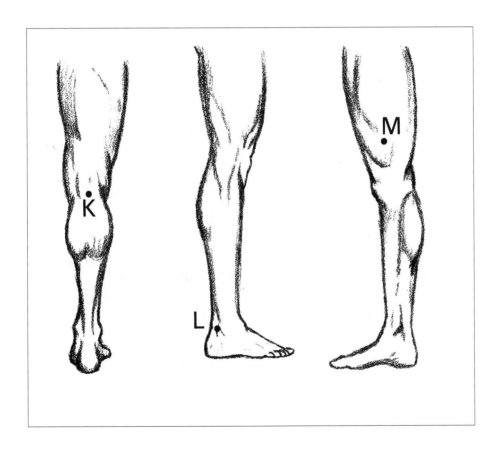

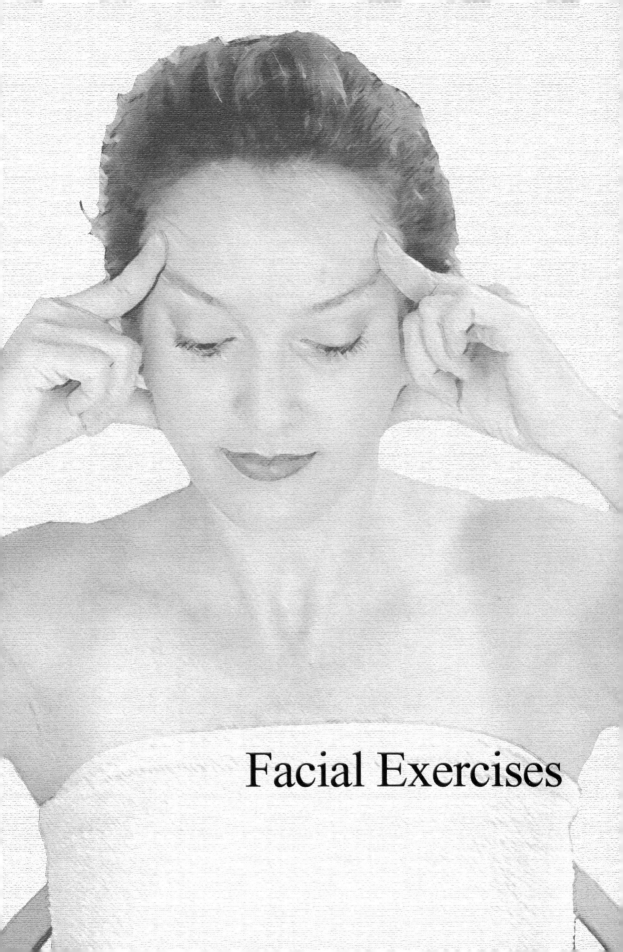

Facial Exercises

The Facial Workout

In many ways facial exercises are like any other type of exercise to keep your body fit. They tone, firm and improve the natural contours of your face. It's like a face lift without the problems and dangers of surgery, and you get superior results that will last a lifetime. We put together eight different exercises for your face. Just like regular body exercises, they work on the principle of resistance to tone and strengthen the muscles. Do them regularly and we guarantee you will see and feel the improvement within a few weeks. Your facial muscles will "firm up" and you will look healthier and more youthful, without having to rely on overpriced exercise books and expensive gadgets.

Exercise #1

Reducing Wrinkles on the Forehead

The *musculus frontalis* is the muscle that lifts the eyebrows and pulls the scalp forward. The habit of lifting the eyebrows creates those wrinkles on the forehead often called "character lines." You'll want to reduce these lines, and to do so you must strengthen this muscle.

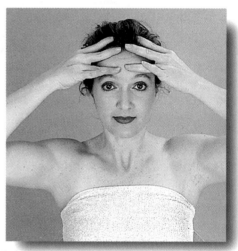

1-A. Place the ring fingers of each hand on the left and right sides of your forehead—not linking, but just touching each other. Next, place the index fingers and thumbs of each hand against the left and right side of the top of your head. Now try to lift your eyebrows against the pressure of your fingers, pulling downward. Do this movement ten times.

1-A.

1-B. Place the index fingers of each hand on the left and right sides of your forehead, with the thumbs just against the jaw line. Push up with your fingers and lift the brow, while at the same time pulling the brow downward, looking down to create as much resistance as possible. Repeat this ten times. Do these exercises regularly, and shortly you will begin noticing a "firming" action taking place. In time you will see a smoother forehead and a softening of "character lines."

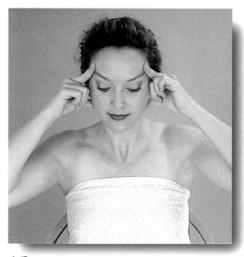

1-B.

Exercise #2

The Eyes and Nose

The *orbicularis oculi* is the muscle that surrounds the entire eye, and opens and closes it. This particular exercise pumps blood into the eye area and strengthens the eyelids. Puffiness, hollowness and deep circles around the eyes, as well as "crow's feet" at the outer edges of the eye area can be diminished. The muscles around the nose are called the *Levator palpebrae superioris* and the *dilator naris anterior.* Since the nose continues to change as we age, becoming wider and dropping, this exercise is very important.

2-A. Place your index fingers on the outside of your eyes and the middle fingers between your eyebrows. Apply pressure, and as you do, close your eyes tightly and squint, drawing your eyebrows inward and downward. This forces wrinkles between the brows, as if you were frowning. You will feel a pulling on your fingers. Then open the eyes as wide as you can, as if you are surprised. Do this ten times.

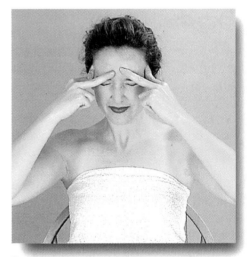

2-A.

2-B. Place the tip of your finger on the end of your nose, then with a firm pressure, shift your mouth to the left as far as you can (as though you're talking out of the corner of your mouth), and then as far to the right as you can. Next, purse your lips as though you're making a mad face, then open your mouth wide (as you would for a dental examination). Do each of these movements ten times.

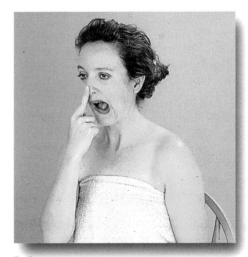

2-B

Exercise #3

The Cheeks

This exercise firms and tones the *buc-cinator* muscle of the cheeks, as well as the *orbicular oris*. Form an open claw with each hand, then place the tips of the fingers over each cheek with the thumbs pressing in on each side of the jaw at the outside ends of the mouth. As you press firmly, open your mouth into a wide "O" shape—as wide as you can—then close the mouth into a "kiss" shape. Do this ten times.

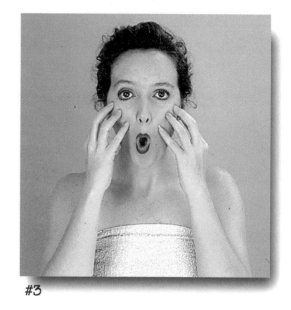

#3

Exercise #4

The Mouth

This exercise tones and strengthens the *zygomaticus* muscle, which tends to droop as we age, and helps prevents a sagging, downwardly turned mouth. Place each index finger at the corners of the mouth. Pressing firmly, pull out-ward on the mouth with your fingers, then purse your lips as if to kiss. This "pull" will force your fingers inward. Smile with lips closed, then purse the lips, repeating this exercise ten times.

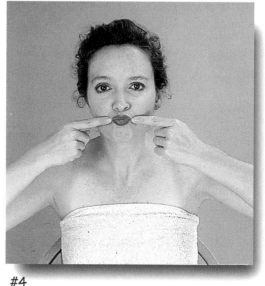

#4

Exercise #5

The Lips

Place the ends of your index fingers in the corners of your mouth, entering the mouth just a fraction of an inch. Press down, then pull with enough pressure to force the lips to expand in a closed mouth smile. Next, pucker the lips so that the fingers are brought inward, then press so that your lips are fixed into an exaggerated pucker. Do this in and out movement ten times.

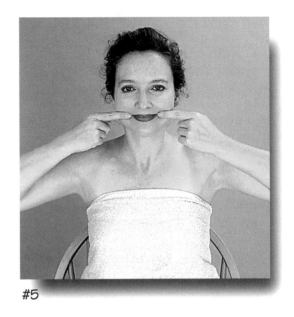

#5

Exercise #6

The Neck

Place your right hand against the right side of your head. Press slightly to offer resistance, then, keeping your eyes looking straight ahead, try to turn your head to the right and look over your right shoulder. Your hand should prevent your head from turning. Then, as though you have lost the battle, allow your right hand to push your head to the left as far as you can. Repeat this same exercise with your left hand on the left side of your head. Do both sides ten times each.

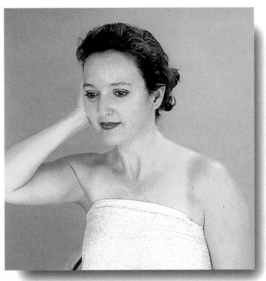

#6

Exercise #7

The Head Roll

When you've completed the neck exercise, do several head rolls by rotating your head in a complete circle to loosen up and relax the neck. Do ten of them.

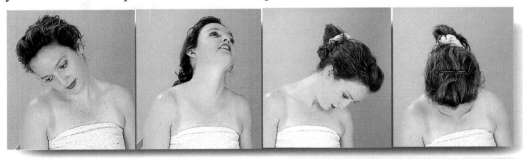

Exercise #8

The Chin and Jaw Line

The *plerygoid internus* muscle in the jaw receives a good workout in this exercise. When strengthened, this muscle prevents droopy jowls and sagging skin.

8-A. Begin with an exaggerated smile, open-mouthed and showing most of your teeth. Actually stretch the smile until you feel a pulling in the neck muscles. As you hold this enormous smile, tilt your head back, then forward as far as you can.

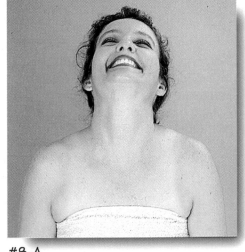

#8-A

8-B. Next lift your head and look straight ahead, then go from the exaggerated smile to a frown. With eyes closed and lips puckered, hold this position tightly until you feel the pull from the muscles in your neck. Then, holding this expression, slowly tilt your head back as far as you can, then forward as far as you can. Do these two moves ten times.

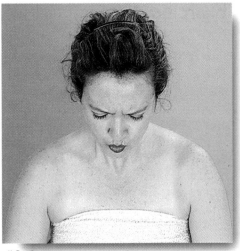

#8-B

Exercise #9

Eliminating a Double Chin

In order to reduce a double chin, you need to strengthen the *musculus mylohyoideus* in the lower jaw.

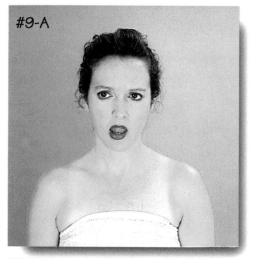

#9-A

9-A. Holding your mouth slightly open, press your tongue against the roof of your mouth. Glide the tongue back as far as it will go inside the mouth, still keeping the tip of your tongue against the roof of your mouth. Slide it back to the front again. Repeat this exercise ten times.

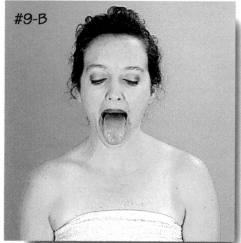

#9-B

9-B. Then open your mouth in an open-mouthed smile and stick your tongue out and downward as far as it will go. Pull the tongue back in and close your mouth. Repeat this movement ten times.

Exercise #10

Firm Up Chin and Neck Area

The *musculus platysma* controls the lower jaw and corners of the mouth. If you exercise this muscle, you will firm up the chin and neck area. Make an open-mouthed (turned down) grimace, pulling this muscle tightly so that you feel the muscles in the neck also pulling and tightening. Hold this expression for a few seconds, then relax your mouth into a normal position. Repeat ten times.

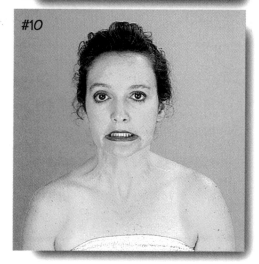

#10

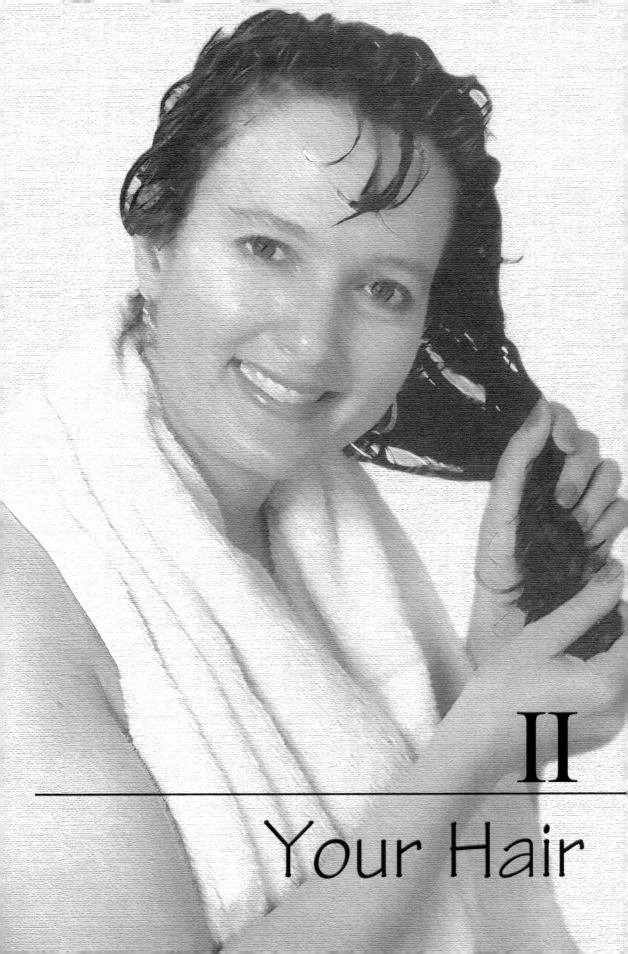

II

Your Hair

The Chemistry of Your Hair

Some cosmetic chemists will tell you that the hair is dead, but nothing could be further from the truth. Each individual hair has its own life cycle, completely independent of that of every other hair. Right at this moment some hairs on your head are actively growing while others are at rest. Eventually, each hair will die and fall out, and will invariably be replaced or not be replaced. Good health, a proper diet and a good hair care system put the odds on your side to get—and keep—a full, lustrous head of hair.

The hair is far more complicated than cosmetic manufacturers and chemists would have you believe, and can be radically affected by both internal (i.e., nutrition) and external (hair care products, sun exposure) factors. The hair shaft is made up of an external layer of overlapping cells known as the cuticle, which is similar to the skin's epidermis in that it has both an outer and an inner coat. The hair cuticle surrounds a mass of spindle-shaped cells known as the paracortex and the orthocortex (see Hair Diagram). As we go deeper, we find a column of superimposed cells called the medulla, which is the innermost section of the hair shaft. The polygon-shaped cells found there are made up of fat granules, air space and the pigment matter that gives hair its color.

The root of each hair contains a bulb which rests on the papilla, through which runs a system of blood vessels responsible for delivering nutrients. Anything that disturbs this pathway destroys the bulb of the hair, causing hair to fall out. Chemical additives in hair care products, as well as certain scalp disorders can disrupt this nourishment process and lead to excessive hair loss and other problems.

The hair follicles are coated with sebum, a complex mixture of lipid substances produced by the sebaceous glands. Sebum is much more than just the oil on your hair. Fatty acids, both saturated and unsaturated, as well as straight-chained and branch-chained molecules (most of which are converted into triglycerides) make up this fatty substance. Sebum is vital to the hair, giving it luster and pliability, and an underproduction of it leads to dry, brittle hair and split ends. Sebum is also responsible for keeping the skin surface around the hair follicles soft and supple. A lack of sebum can result in an accumulation of dead skin cells around the hair follicles, which tend to flake and fall off—dandruff.

The Growth Cycle

The stage at which an individual hair is actively growing is called anagen, and generally lasts from 18 months to several years. The growth takes place when the individual hair cells divide at the sides of the dermal papilla, just below the subcutis (see Hair Diagram). The cells are, at first, very soft and are funneled upward above the region where the hair follicle ceases to be narrow. At this point the cells become hard—or "keratinized"—so they retain their shape for the life of the hair. This anagen, or growth period, dictates the life cycle of the hair—how long the hair will get, and how long it will remain on your head. Most hair never grows more than 36 inches, though some people can grow hair long enough to sit on!

The period when the hair stops growing is called categen. At this point the hair forms a brush-like mass when it is keratinized. During the final stage of the growth cycle, known as telogen, the hair follicle begins to shrink and curl upward into the brush-like mass, where it is held in position and eventually atrophies.

By understanding the hair growth cycle we can begin to understand why proper hair care will complement the natural process of growth, and eliminate the thinning and falling out of hair. Healthy hair is simply a method of keeping the natural hair cycle going. A proper diet, adequate supplementation and mild hair care products free of chemicals and harsh synthetics are ways to extend the life cycle of the hair and keep it full and lustrous. Topical application of certain herbs, vitamins and other nutrients (which we will discuss later) can also be absorbed by the scalp and have been shown to stimulate growth and enhance the health and beauty of your hair.

Massage is another important factor that will encourage the production of new, healthy hair cells. Massaging the scalp during the catagen phase can stimulate hair to grow again, and lightly rubbing the scalp or plucking our the brush-like mass may actually cause hair in both the catagen and telogen phases to grow again. When you shampoo or apply a conditioner or cream rinse to the hair, we strongly recommend that you not only work the treatment through the hair, but that you concentrate on massaging it into your scalp for best results.

Amino Acids and Your Hair

The strength of a human hair is quite surprising. One-on-one, a single hair is stronger than a similarly-sized fiber of aluminum, copper or nylon. This strength comes from the hair's main chemical constituents—amino acids—and their unique chemical arrangement. (See Amino Acids in the Ingredients section of this book.) Eighteen amino acids bond to form the hair protein keratin, which is also present in varying ratios in our skin and nails, and in the wool, horns, hooves and feathers of animals.

The keratin fibers which make up the hair shaft are held together by several different kinds of polypeptide bonds, but the one that gives hair its greatest strength is the disulfide bond formed from the sulfur-containing amino acid cystine, also known as the "cystine bridge." The cystine bridge has one problem, and it's a big one—a number of factors can cause it to break down. Synthetic hair colors destroy it, as do hairsprays with PVP and other copolymers, shampoos made with synthetic detergents, and perm solutions with thioglycolates. Even a hair dryer turned to "hot" can weaken or damage the cystine bridge. When this important bridge that holds the hair shaft together is destroyed or damaged, the hair becomes frayed and starts to look frizzy, split and dull.

Applying the important sulfur-rich amino acids—cystine, cysteine and methionine—directly to the hair has proven extremely effective. Together they work to restore and rebuild the hair shaft from the outside in. That's why using a shampoo, hair conditioner or other hair treatment high in sulfur-containing amino acids may be the best thing you ever do for your hair. We first began introducing amino acids into our hair care products over 30 years ago, combining them with herbs and other nutritional supplements to increase their effectiveness.

Amino acids are also important for the skin, and are an excellent addition to creams and lotions. Indispensable for cellular growth and renewal, they also support

62

the healthy functioning of the sebaceous glands, helping to regulate excessive oil production in both the skin and scalp.

Natural Antidandruff Treatments

The condition known as dandruff can occur at any age in men and women, and its causes differ widely. In most cases, the outer layer of the epidermis of the scalp does not powder off when shed, but tends to clump and form large scales, which are easily visible on the scalp and eventually fall off in flakes. Different factors that can cause dandruff range from hormonal imbalance, diet and stress to increased activity of bacteria and fungi in the scalp, to the use of synthetic or highly alkaline or acid hair care products.

While it is difficult to determine the actual cause of dandruff and other similar scalp conditions, topical application of herbals and other nutrients has been shown to help relieve, control and even eliminate its bothersome symptoms. Commercial antidandruff shampoos contain coal tars and other chemicals that may provide temporary relief, but are harsh and drying to the hair and can be easily absorbed into the body through your scalp. We don't recommend them.

What follows is a list of natural herbs, vitamins and minerals that have been shown to help control and prevent itching and flaking, soothe scalp irritation and promote healing. When buying antidandruff hair care products, look for these ingredients on the labels. Many of the shampoos, conditioners and hair treatments in the Formulas section of this book contain them, either as actual ingredients or as components of an ingredient.

Selenium — This micronutrient mineral high in sulfur-containing amino acids is essential for the health of your scalp. Used in hair formulations for problem hair, it helps remove scalp buildup and control itching and flaking, and makes an excellent natural treatment for dandruff, seborrhea, psoriasis and other scalp conditions. It is the active ingredient in mass produced antidandruff products such as Selsun Blue Shampoo, but you'll find it's much more effective in an all-natural formula. A powerful antioxidant, selenium also helps protect the hair and scalp from sun damage and environmental pollution. It can be slightly drying, so fatty acids and essential oils should be included in formulas containing it.

Sulfur — We've already discussed the value of this important mineral, essential to protein metabolism, which occurs naturally in amino acids and many herbals beneficial to hair and scalp (horsetail and coltsfoot among them). Sulfur can be absorbed into the skin and scalp and incorporated into the keratin of the hair, and hair products containing it can restore damaged hair and aid in reducing scalp problems. Used as an ingredient in shampoos and hair treatments, it should appear on a label as sulfur, biosulfur, or organic sulfur.

B Vitamins (particularly d-Panthenol and Inositol) — The B vitamins are important to the hair and scalp as regulators of the metabolic function and components of an active group of enzymes essential to skin cell respiration. This is vital in the scalp and at the hair bulb, around the dermal papilla. The two most important B vitamins for the hair are d-panthenol and inositol. Regular treatment with products containing panthenol may help improve seborrhea and hair loss. Inositol exerts a favorable influence on the metabolism of the scalp and helps prevent hair damage. Look for these two vitamins in hair care products. (Topical application of B vitamins won't diminish your body's need for B vitamins internally. Taking a good B vitamin complex is still essential for your health.)

Horsetail, Coltsfoot, Nettle — These three herbs are rich in both sulfur and silicic acid. They promote blood flow to the dermal papilla, which nourishes the hair shaft, thereby reducing hair loss and helping control certain scalp conditions. Sometimes referred to as the "hair care trio," we have incorporated these hair-nourishing herbals into many of the hair care formulas in this book, and we suggest you look for products that contain them—but make sure they're all-natural, or the important benefits of these herbs will be greatly reduced. (See Horsetail, Coltsfoot and Nettle in the Ingredients section.)

Rosemary and Sage — Two superb purifiers and hair tonics whose mild antibacterial properties make them ideal in shampoos, conditioners and rinses. Their combined action has been shown to offer relief from the itching, flaking and irritation of many scalp conditions.

Quillaya Bark, Yucca Root, Sarsaparilla Root — These three roots are well known by herbalists for their excellent foaming and cleansing abilities. They offer a superb natural alternative to synthetic detergents used in most commercial shampoos. Quillaya root in particular makes an excellent antidandruff shampoo and also seems to correct the excessive sebum flow brought on by most synthetic detergents.

Cade Tar — Shampoos and soaps containing coal tar were at one time popular antidandruff treatments, but this byproduct of bituminous coal is a strong allergen and very harsh on the hair, scalp and skin. Herbal tar products are far superior. Extracted from cade oil, cade tar is obtained from the distillation of the wood of *Juniperus oxycedrus*, a small tree native to the Mediterranean. Used in hair care preparations for problem scalp and skin, cade tar helps relieve and control the symptoms of eczema, psoriasis and other disorders.

Salicylic Acid — Also known as methyl salicylate, salicylic acid is the main constituent of wintergreen oil, at concentrations of up to 98%. Other natural sources include birch oil, cloves, coca and yarrow. A natural antiinflammatory, analgesic and antiseptic, it is primarily used in hair care products as a treatment for dandruff. One drawback is its strong odor, even when used in small amounts. (Acetylsalicylic acid, a synthetic version of salicylic acid, is more commonly known as aspirin.)

Sweet Bay — An excellent antibacterial and antifungal, this herbal helps prevent flaking and scalp buildup, and is sometimes used in antidandruff shampoos and hair tonics.

Red Squill — Its active principle, called scilliroside, has been found effective in the treatment of dandruff and seborrhea.

Valerian Root — Known for its soothing and calming effect, valerian root also has strong antidandruff properties.

Sketch of a Section of a Hair Fiber

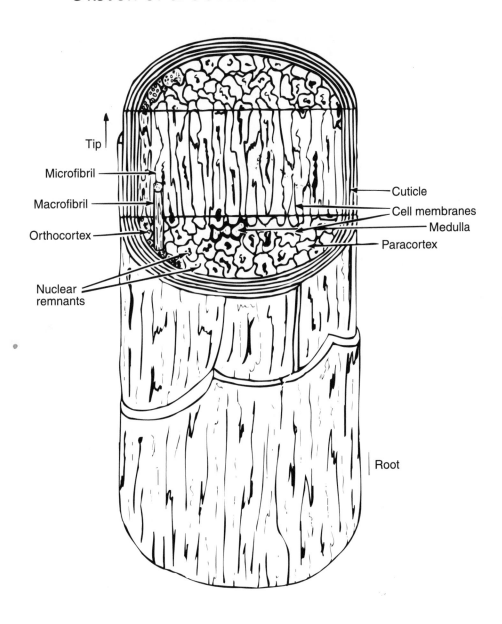

The Take Charge Hair Saver Method

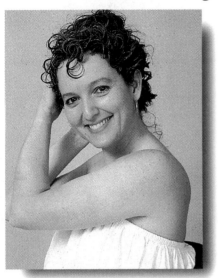

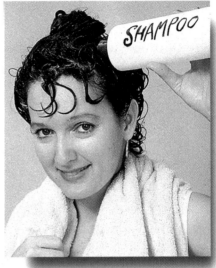

STEP 1 – GREEN HAIR MASK   STEP 2 – SHAMPOO

The natural hair care method discussed here will *save your hair.* These four simple steps using the natural formulas you make yourself will restore the right moisture balance and give you healthier, fuller and more manageable hair by week's end.

STEP 1 — The Hair Mask

This is probably the most important step in your hair care regimen, and the one that will give you the fastest results, particularly if you suffer from thin, lifeless or damaged hair and problem scalp. The Blue Green Algae Hair Rescue Mask (Formula #21) featured here is a deep-conditioning treatment for all hair types, formulated to attract and retain moisture and nourish the hair shaft from the outside in. This "green goop" Priscilla is applying to her hair works wonders on irritated or problem scalp, and will leave your hair soft, full and lustrous from the very first time you use it.

Apply this pre-shampoo mask once or twice a week to dry hair and work it carefully into the scalp and through the hair, making sure to concentrate on the ends. Leave it on for 15 minutes, then rinse off and shampoo as usual.

STEP 2 — Shampoo

This book offers four different shampoos for dry, oily or normal hair and problem scalp. Make the one that works best for your hair type, then use it regularly. Or try a couple of different formulas, and alternate them for best results. Priscilla chose Blue Green Algae Hair Rescue Shampoo for Problem Scalp (Formula #20), the companion shampoo to our hair mask. Apply a small amount of shampoo to wet hair and work well into hair and scalp. Don't worry if the shampoo doesn't lather as well as other mass-produced formulas with heavy synthetic detergents in them. I guarantee your hair is still getting clean. Rinse well in warm water, and repeat if needed.

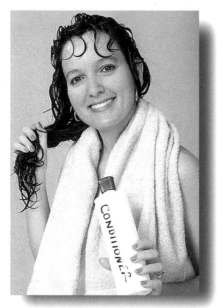
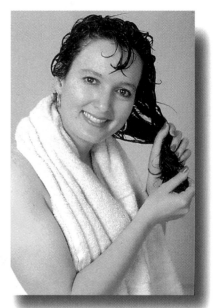

STEP 3— Conditioning

Conditioning is a must for all hair types. A good conditioner restores the right moisture balance to the hair and scalp, smooths out tangles and lightly coats the hair shaft to help repair split ends and add body and shine. If your hair is dry or brittle, you will definitely benefit from a good, protein-rich conditioner like the Jojoba & Aloe Instant Hair Conditioner (Formula #22) Priscilla is using here.

After shampooing, apply a generous amount of conditioner to hair and scalp, then work well into scalp and through hair, concentrating on the ends, particularly if your hair is long or damaged. If your hair is normal, simply use a little less conditioner. Even if your hair tends to be oily, you will still benefit from a good conditioning treatment. If your hair is extra oily, we suggest you shampoo, apply the conditioner, leave it on for five or ten minutes, then shampoo hair again, and rinse thoroughly.

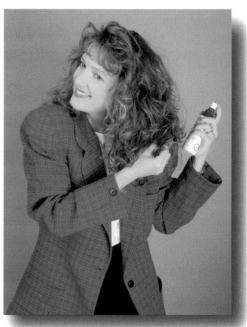

STEP 4— Styling

Styling products are among the worst offenders when it comes to piling chemicals into your hair and scalp. Most hairsprays and gels contain PVP-copolymers, a fancy word for plastic, as well as synthetic alcohols and a long list of other harsh chemicals that can damage the hair

STEP 4 — The Finishing Touch

and be easily absorbed through the scalp.

Here we offer two styling formulas, depending on your hair type and the amount of hair control you need. Our Tangle-Go Luster Spray (Formula #23) is very effective on dry, frizzy or flyaway hair. It contains no herbal gums to "hold" the hair, but simply softens, conditions and helps protect your hair from heat damage due to blow dryers and curling irons. To use, spray it on damp hair before styling, or on dry hair between shampoos to add moisture and shine.

Our White Camellia Amino Acid Hair Spray (Formula #24) is made with amino acids, natural vitamins and herbal gums to nourish and revitalize the hair and provide a light, natural hold (more or less gum arabic may be used for stronger or lighter hair control).

Simply choose the styling formula that's best for your hair type, and use it as often as needed without fear of damaging your hair or polluting the environment with fluorocarbons and other chemicals found in aerosol hairsprays.

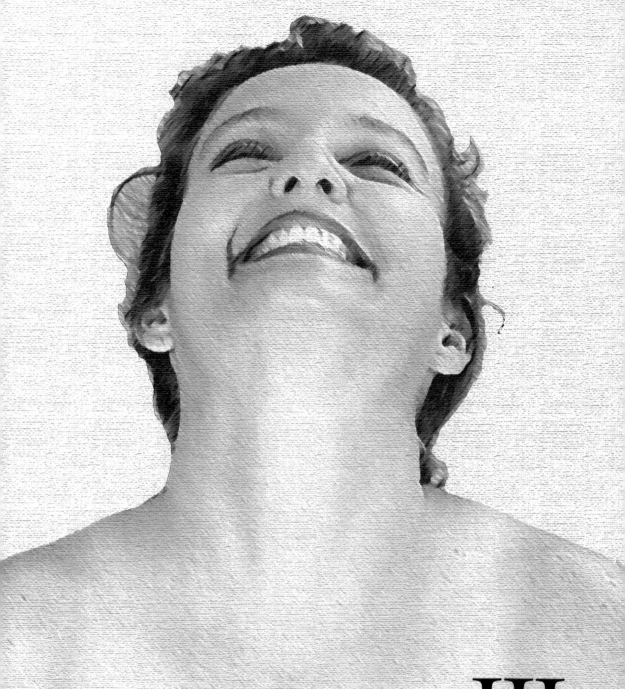

III

Diet, Nutrition and Your Hair & Skin

Y**ou can spend all day in the kitchen** cooking up the most wonderful natural products, or drop a great deal of money at a department store buying the most expensive brand of cosmetics, but if your diet is not what it should be, your hair and skin will show it. Premature wrinkles, rough skin or a sallow, greasy complexion, and dry, brittle hair or a dandruff-prone scalp are some of the problems you can correct with proper nutrition, as well as the right cosmetic products.

The best diet for the health of your hair and skin is based on a simple premise: Eat healthy, balanced meals that avoid anything processed or artificial and emphasize fresh vegetables and fruits. Staying away from hydrogenated or partially-hydrogenated oils, and too many dairy foods, refined grains, sugar and animal products is also a good idea, and will help put you on the right nutrition track.

Vegetables and Fruits: Strive for Five

Though the National Cancer Institute recommends that Americans "strive for five"—that is, eat five servings of fruits and vegetables every day, fewer than 10% of the population actually does. Why the push for produce? Fresh vegetables and fruits are your best protection against degenerative diseases and many forms of cancer because they're high in antioxidants, particularly vitamins A, C and E, and the mineral selenium.

Antioxidants are important to your health because they prevent the formation of free radicals—atoms or groups of atoms that can damage cells and wreak havoc in your body if left unchecked. Here's how the damage happens: Electrons within an atom generally occur in pairs, which makes for a chemically stable arrangement; however, when an electron is unpaired, it is easy for other atoms and molecules to bond with it. Free radicals contain one or more unpaired electrons, which leaves them open to bind with a number of compounds in the body, causing a chemical reaction that can alter the genetic material in the cells and lead to serious cell and tissue damage.

While the presence of a small amount of free radicals in the body is normal, excessive UV ray exposure from the sun and constant contact with toxic chemicals and environmental pollutants (such as cigarette smoke and car exhaust) can cause free radical formation to get out of control. Antioxidants protect the body by binding to free radical electrons, thus neutralizing their cell-damaging action. Free radical damage is believed to be responsible for the body's aging process. It can seriously impair immune system function and lead to a number of illnesses, including type II diabetes, arthritis, heart disease, and particularly, cancer.

According to Gladys Block, Ph.D., professor of epidemiology and nutrition at the University of California at Berkeley School of Public Health, antioxidants in vegetables and fruits offer clear-cut benefits in protecting people from cancer. In 1992 she collected studies published through 1991 that compared diet with cancer rates. Cancers studied included lung, breast, colon, cervical, ovarian, bladder, throat, oral, pancreatic, prostate and stomach—200 studies in total. Every study showed that the greater the amount of fruits and vegetables in the diet, the lower the cancer rate. Those who ate the least amount of fruits and vegetables had twice the cancer rate compared with those who ate the most.

While antioxidants are widely available in a balanced diet high in fruits and vegetables, the less-than-whole foods available in modern markets, coupled with additional stresses on the body caused by pollution and chemicals, make supplementation a smart choice, and one increasingly recommended by physicians everywhere.

The Fat Facts

Nothing in the ordinary American diet has changed more profoundly than the fats we consume daily. Fats are big news right now. Check out any grocery shelf and you'll see fake fat, low fat, trans-fat, saturated fat, no fat, cholesterol-free: you name it, we have a sound bite for it.

Here's the skinny on fat, and of all the diet tips offered in this book, this is the one you'll probably write to thank us for: You need fat. Fat is not bad. The problem is that you are probably eating way too much of the wrong kinds of fat and not nearly enough of the right kinds. The really good news is that changing your bad fat eating habits to good ones will show up on your skin and hair in a fabulous way. Many hair and skin problems you thought were yours for life can become a bad memory if you manage to change your fat eating habits.

Let me give you a little fat history. Sixty years ago our diets were quite different. Most of our food was grown within 100 miles of where we lived, and mass-production of food products was unheard of. Much of the bread and other baked goods we ate was made at home or at a local bakery or small factory. Much of the meat we ate was tougher but leaner, and came from cattle raised on grass, not on grain (which drastically changes the fatty acid ratio of the meat from unsaturated to saturated). We ate more vegetables, grains and beans because meat was expensive, and was used more as a flavoring than as a main course. We ate butter, not margarine, in which we fried our eggs, which came from chickens that scratched in our own backyards. Every one of the above facts points to a healthier time in our fat consumption history.

One important change in our diet came with the development of factory farming, which supplies the majority of the meat and poultry and much of the seafood we eat today. Structured around the bottom line, factory farming grows unhealthy, drugged and obese animals raised on pesticide-contaminated feed and large quantities of antibiotics and hormones. These are passed on to us in their meat and eggs, which are much less wholesome than the animal foods our grandparents ate.

According to David Steinman and Samuel S. Epstein, M.D. (*The Safe Shopper's Bible,* Macmillan, 1995), 40 of the animal drugs and pesticides presently known to be found as residues in meat and poultry are carcinogenic, and as many as 4,000 new drugs used on animals could have serious adverse effects on both animals and humans. Growth-stimulating hormones (listed as known carcinogens by the International Agency for Research on Cancer) are also administered to over 90% of the cattle raised for slaughter, posing another serious threat to our health whenever we bite into a hamburger or crack another egg into the frying pan.

The growth of the vegetable oil industry is another important factor that has influenced our consumption of fat. Sixty years ago, only unrefined vegetable oils and animal fats were used in baking and cooking. Today, with the development of hydrogenated oils, these unhealthy but shelf-stable fats can be found in nearly all commercially available baked or processed foods.

You see, unrefined vegetable oils are fragile, full of highly unsaturated fatty acids that can become rancid fairly quickly. As a result, the rapidly expanding vegetable oil industry developed high-heat processing and hydrogenation, which extend the shelf-life of the oils. These processes biochemically change oils from nutritious to nasty. Here's how: in its fresh, unprocessed state, a polyunsaturated fatty acid chain is in the *cis*-formation. This means there are hydrogen atoms attached on just one side of the molecule. The molecule then "kinks" because the hydrogen atoms repel one another, forming a spiral. If the fatty acids are subjected to hydrogenation, then the molecule "unkinks," and the hydrogen atoms relocate to either side of the molecule. This causes the liquid oil to become solid—think margarine—and the fatty acids are said to be in the *trans*-formation.

The problem is that trans-fatty acids cannot be used by the body as effectively as cis-fatty acids. Yet fat is vital for many body processes. For instance, every cell membrane contains fat. Both brain and nerve tissue are very high in fat. The skin, nails and hair all require fat to maintain structural integrity. The stomach requires fat to maintain a healthy lining; thus, good fat nutrition can prevent digestive problems of all sorts.

Fat is also a precursor to the production of prostaglandins, hormones that control many body functions. Because the typical Western diet is high in animal foods, one series of prostaglandins (PG2) is often overproduced; this is the series responsible for inflammation, blood clotting and water retention—a few of the symptoms of many modern degenerative diseases. The overproduction of PG2 is a sign of our imbalanced fat consumption. Furthermore, two series of prostaglandins—PG1 and PG3—which work to reduce inflammation, water retention and excessive clotting while increasing immune function, are underproduced if you eat too many of the wrong kinds of fats.

The fat necessary for these important processes cannot be manufactured by the body. For that reason, these nutrients are called the essential fatty acids (EFA's), which must be obtained from the diet. The problem is that when not enough EFA's are present, the body must make do with trans-fatty acids, and the results can be less than satisfactory.

Here's an example: fat is essential in maintaining healthy blood vessels, which are constantly transporting and exchanging nutrients with surrounding cells. But bad fat nutrition means that blood vessels don't have adequate EFA's to maintain healthy membranes. As a result, the body manufactures cholesterol and adhesive proteins to repair membranes. Over the years, this sort of "jerry-rigged" repair of blood vessels may well lead to arteriosclerosis, the primary symptom of cardiovascular disease. Changing your fat nutrition from bad to good, and increasing the amount of antioxidants you get in your diet through fruits and vegetables will greatly reduce your chances of ever getting heart disease, as well as giving you healthy, beautiful skin and hair.

As you can see, good fat nutrition means you must think of fat as an important part of your everyday diet, but you must choose your fats wisely. The fats present in animal foods are largely saturated, and saturated fats, blamed for many degenerative diseases, will do more harm than good.

While it is true that the consumption of animal foods has increased over the past 60 years, these degenerative diseases are not simply caused by too much meat in your diet or by ingesting too many hydrogenated and partially-hydrogenated vegetable oils. With the meteoric rise in the overconsumption of these bad fats has come the underconsumption of the good fats, the essential fatty acids. According to Edward Siguel, M.D., Ph.D., author of *Essential Fatty Acids in Health and Disease* (Nutrek Press, 1994), a deficiency of EFA's has been linked to over 60 diseases, including obesity, arthritis, cancer, autoimmune and heart diseases, type II diabetes, premature aging, and Parkinson's and Alzheimer's diseases. Furthermore, of all the nutritional factors vital for good health (which add up to around 50), the EFA's are required in greater quantity than any other, and should make up approximately eight to nine percent of your total calorie intake (though you may consume more with no harm).

The most important essential fatty acids are linoleic acid, also known as an Omega-6 fatty acid for its chemical structure, and alpha-linolenic acid, an Omega-3 fatty acid. These EFA's are available in a wide variety of unprocessed foods, but the source we're going to recommend is flaxseed oil, although not just any flaxseed oil. Flaxseed oil is fantastically fragile: it is so reactive to oxygen and light that if left unrefrigerated for less than an hour, it develops a rancid "skin." For best results, you must purchase organic, cold-pressed, refrigerated flaxseed oil in brown glass or opaque black plastic bottles, clearly marked with a pressing date and a "use-by" date.

We cannot emphasize too strongly how important it is to consume only fresh flaxseed oil: if the oil tastes bitter or rancid, then you are consuming lipid peroxides, which are quite harmful to the body. Fresh flaxseed oil has a delicious, nutty flavor; keep it refrigerated at all times. If you are now healthy, then one tablespoon will help you maintain. If your skin is dry, or your cholesterol high, then we recommend you take at least two tablespoons per day. Feel free to combine flaxseed oil with herbs and vinegar for an exquisite salad dressing, or pour a little over steamed vegetables. (Do not sauté with this oil, however, as heating it will destroy the nutrients.)

If you are counting your calories and fat grams, remember this: flaxseed oil will not make you gain weight; quite the contrary. It will help stimulate your metabolism so that you can lose weight. Because the EFA's in this wonderful oil are so vital to nutrition, your body will use up this fat quickly instead of storing it.

Taking EFA's is only part of the battle; the other part is eliminating the bad fat in your diet. You must stop eating all foods containing trans-fatty acids. Throw out the margarine, and read the labels on all store-bought baked goods and processed foods—anything with the words "partially hydrogenated" printed on the label must go! Evaluate your consumption of saturated fat, which includes all meat and dairy products. Be sure that the animal products you eat are low-fat, and try to buy organic. The reason for this is that pesticides and other synthetic chemical residues tend to build up in fat (remember how many harmful chemicals can dissolve in fat). You'll want to avoid these to keep from getting residues building up in your fat.

Once you've taken steps to improve your fat nutrition, here are some benefits you can expect within four to six weeks: If your skin is dry and scaly, there will be a noticeable difference in texture—you will literally feel your hands and feet becoming softer. If you have oily skin, it will begin to look and feel much less greasy, particularly in the T-zone areas of the nose and chin. Long-standing eczema may improve. You will have more energy but be calm, less reactive to stressful situations. You will not gain weight. And the next time you have a physical, you may be in for a pleasant surprise: lower cholesterol, lower blood pressure, and higher HDL (the so-called "good" cholesterol).

Buy Organic

In the 1996 edition of *Vital Signs* (published by the Worldwatch Institute), one of the few encouraging statistics is the growth of organic agriculture in the United States. Amid the grim figures that show an increase in global warming, auto emissions, human rights abuses and infectious diseases, are the cheerful statistics that organic agriculture consumption and production are on the upswing. Considering that as many as 30 different pesticides can be used on strawberries alone (according to the Environmental Working Group, a Washington, D.C.-based consumer group), this is good news indeed!

There's little doubt that exposure to pesticides can damage the immune system and cause neurological problems. One of the most troubling areas of research is how pesticide exposure can affect future generations, both through infertility and damaged DNA. These potent chemicals are able to damage the body's inner workings because they belong to a class of chemicals known as "endocrine disrupters." These chemicals, which are by no means limited to pesticides but also include PCBs and dioxin, mimic and displace the role of hormones in the body. Studies indicate it is possible that endocrine-disrupting chemicals may be linked to lower sperm counts, damaged thyroid development, attention deficit disorder, and diseases of the reproductive system, including breast and prostate cancer. Forty percent of pesticides used in agriculture are known or suspected endocrine disrupters.

Around half of all fruits and vegetables go to market with pesticide residues, and 40% have multiple residues. The good news, however, is that grains and low fat dairy products usually contain fewer pesticide residues than produce. This is due to how grain is grown and processed, and where pesticides tend to be stored in animals, including humans: in the liver and fatty tissues.

Avoiding high fat animal products can protect you from pesticide exposure, but one sure way is to buy organic dairy products, which are widely available in health food stores. Avoiding imported produce may also protect you, as the FDA (Food and Drug Administration) is able to examine only about one percent of all lots of foods from abroad, where pesticide residues have been measured at three times the level of a domestically-grown crop. Fruits and vegetables from South America and Mexico are particularly at risk, as pest management on crops in warmer climates relies on heavy application of pesticides, many of which are banned from use in the United States.

If you can't afford to purchase all organic produce, or if it's not available in your area, the previously mentioned Environmental Working Group (EWG) can help you choose which fruits and vegetables are most free from pesticide residues. The EWG examined FDA inspection data between 1992 and 1993, and rated 42 vegetables for pesticide residue content. Their recommendations: buy certified organic strawberries, since the residues in America's favorite red berry are by far the highest of the group, and more than a third of the lots examined contained two or more pesticides. Fortunately, many of the vegetables most recommended for good health—cauliflower, sweet potatoes, cabbages, carrots, bananas and broccoli—were all at the healthy end of the list for pesticide residues. (EWG's complete report, *A Shopper's Guide to Pesticides in Produce,* is available on the Internet at http://www.ewg.org.)

Supplements: Choosing Wisely

There is no doubt that nutritional deficiencies can show on your skin. One of the most notorious examples is pellagra, a disease caused by a niacin deficiency, which in its early stages is characterized by an itchy, red rash. (In fact, pellagra, which reached epidemic proportions in 18th century Italy and Spain, means "rough skin" in Italian.) It is known that an insufficiency of any of the following nutrients— vitamin A, B vitamins, vitamin E and zinc—can cause dermatitis. Fortunately, proper supplementation of these and other vitamins and nutrients will prevent or reduce many skin problems, including acne, premature wrinkles and damage to the skin caused by too much sun exposure.

Beta Carotene and Vitamin A

Beta carotene, the substance that makes carrots and cantaloupes orange, is the most studied member of the carotenoid family. It easily converts in the body to vitamin A, which is very beneficial to your skin. Beta carotene supplementation is considered safer, as even a little too much vitamin A—only 10,000 IU—has been linked to birth defects, while 50,000 IU, taken regularly, can damage the liver and spleen, cause anemia, joint stiffness and pain, and even make your hair fall out. Do we have your attention yet? Don't overdo this one.

However, in the right doses, vitamin A is very important to your skin and hair. It helps regulate sebum production in the skin and scalp, which makes it an essential part of treating acne or overly-oily skin and hair. (Zinc is also necessary for the utilization of vitamin A by the body, so be sure your diet includes adequate zinc.)

Both beta carotene and vitamin A are vital to building and maintaining an effectively-functioning immune system. Plus, vitamin A is an antioxidant, which means it helps reduce free radical damage to your body. Good food sources of these nutrients are deep green or yellow vegetables and fruits, such as sweet potatoes, carrots, pumpkins and other winter squash, cantaloupes, mangoes, dandelion, turnip and beet greens. Recommended daily amount: 5,000 IU vitamin A or 15,000 IU beta-carotene.

B-Complex Vitamins

The B-complex vitamins are the essential "cogs" in all your cells, so they're vital to the health of your entire body, including the skin and hair. B vitamins are used in energy production and help maintain a healthy nervous system and good brain function. For best absorption, the B-Complex vitamins should be taken together, but additional supplementation of certain B vitamins may be necessary for specific disorders. Let's look at these important nutrients individually.

Thiamine (Vitamin B-1)

Thiamine promotes circulation and proper blood formation, and has an active role in the formation of hydrochloric acid, essential for digestion. Though thiamine deficiency is relatively rare today, this vitamin was discovered for its role in alleviating beriberi, once common in Asia because of the high amounts of white rice consumed there. However, thiamine deficiency may occur today among elderly people, alcoholics and epileptics who are taking the prescription drug Dilantin. Mild deficiencies may result in depression, fatigue, insomnia and nerve dysfunction.

Good food sources include nutritional yeast, wheat germ, sunflower seeds, pine nuts, peanuts with skins, soybeans, Brazil nuts, pecans, beans and peas. Recommended daily allowance: 50 mg., taken as part of a B vitamin complex or a multivitamin-mineral formula.

Riboflavin (Vitamin B-2)

Recent research indicates that this B vitamin has antioxidant properties and is an integral part of the chemical process that produces glutathione, an important protector of cells against free radical damage. Oily, scaly skin, surface blood vessels and whiteheads, as well as chapped lips and cracks in the corners of the mouth, are all signs that riboflavin supplementation might be helpful. Because of poor nutrition and decreased ability to absorb vitamins, low levels of riboflavin may occur in older people and some vegans. Alcohol and birth control pills can also interfere with the body's ability to absorb this vitamin. Signs of deficiency include light sensitivity, trembling of hands, dizziness, insomnia, watery and bloodshot eyes, and numbness or burning of the hands and feet. Good food sources for riboflavin include nutritional yeast, liver, almonds, wheat germ, wild rice, mushrooms, poultry and fish. Recommended daily allowance: 20 mg., taken as part of a B vitamin complex or a multivitamin-mineral formula.

Niacin (Vitamin B-3)

Essential for good blood circulation and healthy skin, as well as for proper function of the nervous system, niacin is helpful in preventing headaches, depression, insomnia, bad breath, swollen and painful gums and digestive problems. Recent research notes that niacin supplementation may help lower cholesterol levels and ease the symptoms of arthritis. Combined with immunosuppressive drugs, it has been used to treat recently-diagnosed, insulin-dependent diabetics with impressive results.

NOTE: Because niacin releases histamine, which dilates blood vessels on the skin, a "niacin flush" may result when taking more than 50 mg. of this supplement. Other mild side effects may include tingling, a "hot" feeling and a red cast to the skin, as if you were sunburned. This should go away in 15 to 20 minutes and is not harmful. To reduce the "flush" effect, take your niacin supplement with food or a cold beverage. Inositol hexaniacinate and niacinamide are forms of niacin which will not produce this "flush" reaction when taken.

Good food sources for this vitamin include nutritional yeast, brown rice, wheat bran and peanuts with skins. Recommended daily allowance: 80 mg. niacinamide.

Pantothenic Acid (Vitamin B-5, Panthenol)

Long considered the "antistress vitamin" for its role in supporting adrenal function, pantothenic acid is widely available in food and food supplements, notably calcium pantothenate and pantethine (its most active form). Not enough pantothenic acid in the diet can lead to fatigue, numbness and shooting pains in the feet, but deficiencies of this B vitamin are not common; in fact, its name comes from the Greek word pantos, which means "everywhere."

The skin responds very well to topical applications of pantothenic acid, as do the hair and scalp. A natural hydrator, it also acts as a hair thickener, used in hair sprays and gels to add body and moisture to thin, lackluster hair. When added to creams and lotions, it is an excellent humectant, attracting moisture to the skin. We use a natural form of pantothenic acid—panthenol—in many of our hair and skin care products.

Good food sources for pantothenic acid include nutritional yeast, liver, peanuts, mushrooms, split peas, pecans and soybeans. Recommended daily allowance: 50 mg., taken as part of a B vitamin complex or a multivitamin-mineral formula.

Pyridoxine (Vitamin B-6)

This water-soluble B vitamin is involved in more bodily functions than any other nutrient. Sixty enzymes depend on it for proper functioning, including one that regulates normal cross-linking of collagen and elastin, two of the main proteins found in the skin. Pyridoxine provides a degree of immunity against cancer and helps prevent arteriosclerosis and some forms of heart disease by inhibiting the formation of homocysteine, a toxic substance that can adversely affect the heart muscle and blood vessels. It also plays an important role in the balance of female hormones, and acts as a mild diuretic, providing relief from premenstrual syndrome. Because birth control pills deplete the supply of this vitamin, women who take them may suffer from a mild B-6 deficiency, which could lead to depression, irritability, tiredness and erratic mood changes. A deficiency can also cause eczema and seborrhea, and cracking around the lips.

Because vitamin B-6 requires magnesium to be used by the body, any supplementation should include this mineral. Toxic reactions have been reported with amounts as low as 150 mg. per day, so only take high dosages of this vitamin under a physician's supervision.

Good food sources include nutritional yeast, sunflower seeds, wheat germ, walnuts, lentils, bananas and Brussels sprouts. Recommended daily allowance: 50 mg., taken as part of a B vitamin complex or a multivitamin-mineral formula.

Vitamin B-12 (Cobalamin)

This is one supplement every vegetarian should take, as this vitamin occurs only in animal foods. (Though a form of vitamin B-12 is present in fermented soybean products and seaweed, it may not be the appropriate form our bodies need.) Further, as this vitamin is stored primarily in the liver and kidneys, and such small amounts are necessary (the RDA is only 2 mcg.), deficiency symptoms may take up to six years to show up. The classic one for this vitamin is pernicious anemia, but impaired neurological and nerve function also can occur, particularly among the elderly, whose ability to absorb this nutrient may be impaired due to poor digestion. Vitamin B-12 supplementation has been found to be helpful in treating AIDS, Alzheimer's, depression, asthma, diabetic neuropathy, low sperm counts, multiple sclerosis and tinnitus.

Good food sources for vitamin B-12 include liver and other organ meats, clams, oysters, sardines, trout, salmon, fresh tuna, dried whey and many cheeses. Recommended daily allowance: 100 mcg. daily, taken as part of a B vitamin complex or a multivitamin-mineral formula.

Biotin

This very important vitamin is closely linked to the health of the skin, scalp and nails, and its deficiency shows up quickly. Flaking, itching and irritation and weak, brittle nails can often be prevented with proper supplementation, as biotin is critical to the metabolic process that produces keratin, the main protein found in the hair, skin and nails. A recent Swiss study determined that people who took 2,500 mcg. of biotin found their nails became 25% thicker. This essential nutrient is often added to skin care formulas and hair growth products with excellent results.

Because biotin is an expensive ingredient, look for at least 25 mcg. in a multivitamin, suggests Michael Castleman in his recent book, *Nature's Cures*. Less than that indicates the manufacturer may be skimping.

Good food sources of biotin include brewer's yeast, peanuts, walnuts, egg yolks, cauliflower, molasses, milk, corn and barley. Be sure to look for it in unprocessed foods, as canning and heat curing destroy this nutrient. Recommended daily allowance: 300 mcg.

Folic Acid

A known brain food, folic acid is necessary for protein metabolism, proper immune system function and the production of red blood cells. A deficiency of this important B vitamin often manifests itself as chapped lips and cracked skin at the corners of the mouth, but health problems from not getting enough folic acid can last a lifetime.

Recent discoveries show it to be absolutely vital in preventing birth defects. Early in pregnancy, the brain and the spinal cord of the embryo close, forming a continuous structure. Deficiency of folic acid can cause this neural tube to fail to close, which can lead to spina bifida, hydrocephalus and other congenital defects. Even more recently, folic acid was discovered to be one of the three B vitamins responsible for keeping the homocysteine levels low in your blood. Homocysteine is an artery-attacking amino acid that may be high in the bloodstreams of people who eat meat. These high levels result from an inability to convert the amino acid methionine into cysteine. High levels of homocysteine cause arteriosclerosis, and may be responsible for up to 50% of all heart attacks.

Folic acid is widely available in food as folate; however, it may be difficult to absorb in this form, according to noted alternative physician Dr. Julian Whitaker. Also, the use of common medications such as aspirin, birth control pills, estrogen and antacids can increase your need for folic acid. Good food sources for folic acid include asparagus, Brussels sprouts, spinach, broccoli, and pinto and navy beans. Recommended daily allowance: 400 mcg.

Vitamin C

From curing the common cold to eradicating wrinkles, this vitamin is a major player in the world of nutrition. In fact, some nutritionists credit the recent improvements in heart disease statistics to increased supplementation with this inexpensive, popular vitamin. Its role in skin care is twofold: first, its primary function is the manufacture of collagen; second, it is the main water-soluble antioxidant used by the body. Supplementation with vitamin C can reduce the damage to the body—and the skin—from oxidation and chemical pollution.

The importance of vitamin C to the health of your skin cannot be overstated. However, this vitamin superstar has been shown to be highly beneficial in either treating or preventing a number of other disorders. People (particularly children) suffering from asthma—whose numbers have been on the increase by over 40%—seem to experience fewer symptoms when they supplement their diet with vitamin C. The connection between vitamin C and heart disease has also been well documented. Numerous studies have shown that this amazing supplement helps prevent—even reverse—heart disease by reducing oxidative damage to low-density lipoprotein (LDL), while strengthening the collagen of the arterial walls, lowering cholesterol and blood pressure, and raising high density lipoprotein (HDL). Whew!

Vitamin C's role in cancer prevention is undeniable. Epidemological studies have demonstrated that the lower the vitamin C intake, the higher the rate of cancer. The rates of cancers of the breast, cervix, colon, esophagus, lung and pancreas are lowered with vitamin C supplementation, and cancer patients treated with 10 grams of vitamin C daily appeared to have a longer survival rate, according to two studies by Dr. Ewan Cameron. Cataracts and macular degeneration—the two major causes of blindness among older Americans—can be reduced with vitamin C supplementation.

Like heart disease, diabetes is another degenerative disorder that can be helped with a healthy dose of vitamin C. Many of the symptoms of diabetes, in fact, resemble those of vitamin C deficiency—poor wound healing, fragile capillaries and a depressed immune system among them. One reason for this deficiency, even when diabetics consume foods high in vitamin C, is that insulin helps carry this vitamin into the cells. Since most diabetics suffer from insufficient or inefficient insulin production and function, vitamin C levels can also be too low. Many nutritionists recommend that diabetics take three or more grams of this vitamin daily.

Since vitamin C levels in seminal fluids are higher than in other body fluids, it should come as no surprise that infertility among men also appears to be lessened with supplements of this remarkable substance. Sperm count and motility are improved after vitamin C is added to the diet.

Vitamin C is also vital to the manufacture of healthy collagen. As the body's most important antioxidant, it helps neutralize free radicals in the skin and boosts the immune system by aiding in detoxification through stimulation of the growth and function of white blood cells. According to Michael Murray, vitamin C is similar to interferon, the body's natural antiviral and anticancer compound.

Everyone has heard how vitamin C can "cure" the common cold, or at least lessen its symptoms and its duration. Vitamin C helps reduce the amount of histamine in the blood, which causes the improvement in itchy, watery eyes and runny noses. You can heal yourself from a severe cold with nothing more than large doses of vitamin C—which brings me to the question of dosage:

How much vitamin C is enough, and how much is too much? Linus Pauling (the Nobel Prize-winning doctor who made Vitamin C a household word) estimated his vitamin C intake by comparing human and animal metabolism, since most animals can manufacture vitamin C in their bodies, but humans—along with monkeys—cannot. Dr. Pauling estimated that for his size, weight and age, he would need 18 grams of vitamin C daily. On the other hand, the RDA for vitamin C is a mere 60 mg.

We know Vitamin C is extremely safe, even in very high doses. And you use more vitamin C when you're tired, stressed, under the weather, or have been exposed to toxic substances. Diarrhea and gas may occur if you're taking too much vitamin C; simply take less if these problems develop.

Good food sources for vitamin C include red and green sweet peppers, kale and collard greens, broccoli, Brussels sprouts, watercress, strawberries, oranges and grapefruit. Recommended daily allowance: 3,000 grams vitamin C (buffered with calcium), taken in two divided doses.

Vitamin E

Dubbed the "anti-sterility" vitamin when it was first discovered over 70 years ago, vitamin E (or d-alpha tocopherol) is most well known today for its antioxidant protective qualities. As you increase your intake of polyunsaturated fats (such as flaxseed oil), you will need to take more of this vitamin, which protects fats from oxidation, an extremely important job. In fact, vitamin E's primary role is to maintain the integrity of cellular membranes, protecting them from heavy metals, toxic compounds, drugs, radiation and free radicals. As the most important fat-soluble antioxidant, vitamin E helps prevent three of America's most prevalent "killer" diseases: heart disease, cancer and strokes. Supplementation has also proved invaluable in treating acne, fibrocystic breast disease, menopause, osteoarthritis, eczema, menopause and PMS.

Though vitamin E is a fat-soluble vitamin, supplementation is extremely safe, even at high dosages. Vitamin E is measured in "international units," or IUs. Be sure to take only natural vitamin E (listed as d-alpha tocopherol or d-alpha tocopheryl acetate or succinate) on the label. The synthetic form of vitamin E, listed as dl-alpha, is not as effective and may inhibit the body's ability to absorb natural vitamin E. Look also for mixed tocopherols. Although the other tocopherols—a-beta, d-gamma and d-delta—have not been nearly as extensively studied as d-alpha, evidence is mounting that they are also important in protecting health. Since all the tocopherols are found together in nature, it may be that they function better when taken together.

Good food sources for vitamin E include unrefined polyunsaturated vegetable oils, seeds, nuts and whole grains. Recommended daily allowance: 800 IU mixed tocopherols (including tocotrienols).

Calcium

The role of calcium in the prevention of osteoporosis has been widely publicized, but this important mineral has many other valuable functions. Besides helping form healthy bones and teeth, calcium acts as a regulator of nerve and muscle function, heartbeat, blood clotting and cholesterol levels, and plays an active part in preventing cardiovascular disease.

A stable level of calcium is of vital importance, and in order to maintain this balance in the body, the necessary calcium is "borrowed" from the bones, where 99% of the mineral is stored. Thus, a calcium deficiency can lead to bone loss and a host of other problems. A lack of calcium can also be responsible for aching joints, muscle cramps, high blood pressure, heart palpitations and insomnia, as well as tooth decay, brittle nails, eczema and a dull, pasty complexion.

If you're getting calcium from your diet, dairy foods are still your best bet, with one cup of nonfat yogurt containing 450 mg. However, according to noted vegan physician Dr. Neal Barnard, author of *Food for Life*, a diet too high in protein can cause unabsorbed calcium to be excreted in the urine. Countries where dairy products are most consumed also have the highest rates of hip fracture, a statistic that seems to support this view. While vegans used to be criticized for a lack of calcium in their diet, we now know this vital nutrient is widely available from plant sources, including kale (170 mg. per cup) and tofu (517 mg. per cup).

If you use a calcium supplement, remember to take it with food and in amounts not exceeding 500 mg. at one time. Authorities differ as to which form of calcium is most easily absorbed with fewest side effects. One problem with calcium supplements, according to Dr. Julian Whitaker, is that they can interfere with the absorption of other minerals. His recommendation: calcium citrate. To be absorbed, calcium needs adequate amounts of vitamin D and magnesium. Other good food sources for calcium include greens, canned salmon or sardines with bones and corn tortillas processed with lime. Recommended daily allowance: 1,000 mg. (in 500 mg. increments, twice daily).

Iron

Splitting nails? Then perhaps your problem is too little iron in your diet. Cold hands and feet and a sore tongue are other possible symptoms. Yet excessive iron supplementation has been linked to more deaths than any other nutrient. The reason: you need a little iron to manufacture hemoglobin, but not too much, and this mineral is readily available in foods, particularly meat. Here's one time when the experts agree that the RDA (recommended daily allowance) is enough, and not to exceed it. Many food supplements don't include iron, as it can interfere with the absorption of other nutrients.

Good food sources for iron include beef, baked potatoes, pumpkin seeds, clams and soybeans. Recommended daily allowance: 18 mg.

Magnesium

One of the most studied minerals, magnesium is essential in a variety of vital processes. It is a cofactor in over 100 enzyme reactions in the body, including the all-important absorption of calcium. Necessary for heart health, it is used to lower blood pressure and prevent heart attacks. A low level of magnesium can be an indication of someone predisposed to migraines or premenstrual syndrome.

Insufficient consumption of magnesium is extremely common. Some researchers estimate up to 40% of Americans consume too little magnesium. Furthermore, many prescription drugs, including asthma medications, diuretics, Digitalis and other cardiovascular medications, as well as alcohol, caffeine and stress all remove magnesium from the body.

Good food sources for magnesium include brown rice, oatmeal, avocados, spinach, haddock, baked potatoes, navy and lima beans, broccoli, yogurt and bananas. Recommended daily allowance: 500 mg.

Potassium

This mineral is present in the body in the form of an electrolyte, a mineral salt that conducts electricity. Electrolytes help balance water distribution, pH, and muscle, nerve, heart, kidney and adrenal functions, and help regulate chemical reactions within the cells.

There are three types of electrolytes—potassium, sodium and chloride—which must occur in the right balance in the body. However, due to an emphasis on processed foods, the standard American diet tends to be twice as heavy in sodium and chloride (in the form of common table salt) as it is in potassium, which is widely present in fruits and vegetables. An imbalance in potassium-sodium consumption is implicated in many diseases, including cancer and heart conditions.

A potassium deficiency—which can occur from too much exercise, vomiting or diarrhea—can be very debilitating. Symptoms include mental confusion, irritability, weakness, heart disturbances, muscle cramps, loss of appetite, insomnia and nerve conduction problems. Many nutritionists recommend supplementing potassium and magnesium together.

Good food sources of potassium include bananas, avocado, lima beans, peaches, chicken, cod, flounder and salmon. Recommended daily allowance: up to 5.6 grams per day, especially for athletes, the elderly and people with high blood pressure.

Flavonoids

Flavonoids are plant pigments that give fruits and flowers their colors, but recent research has shown they may also be beneficial in treating or preventing many diseases. While not exactly vitamins, they are essential to good health, as they make vitamins, particularly vitamin C, work more effectively. In addition, many are potent antioxidants, effective against viruses, cancer-causing agents, excessive cholesterol and diabetic complications.

While more than 4,000 flavonoids have been identified, we find two types to be particularly beneficial for the skin. PCO (procyanidolic oligomers) was first studied for its ability to strengthen capillaries and veins, but a greater benefit may lie in its strong antioxidant properties, which are greater than those of vitamins C and E. This nutrient is an important part of skin care, as it helps protect skin from UV damage, and also helps prevent the attack of skin proteins by free radicals and inflammation.

Green tea polyphenols, most notably the tongue-twisting constituent *Epigallocatechin gallate* (a flavonoid), possess antioxidant activity 20 times greater than vitamin E, and some credit them for the excellent longevity of the Japanese people, who are heavy drinkers of green tea. Clinical studies have shown that green tea, when applied to the skin, does appear to reduce the incidence of skin cancer, as well as free radical damage. We use powdered Matcha green tea from Japan in many of our cosmetic products, but green tea leaves (organic), available from your health food store, offer many of the same properties and are easier to obtain. Keep your eyes peeled for cosmetics containing green tea, including some of the recipes on the Formulas section of this book. Whether consumed as a beverage or applied to the skin, green tea is a fantastically healthy food.

Other good food sources of flavonoids include citrus fruits, berries, onions, parsley and red wine. Another excellent supplementation source of flavonoids is grape seed extract. Recommended daily allowance: 100 mg. grape seed extract. Also, we urge you to sip at least two cups of green tea daily.

Selenium

This trace—but absolutely vital—mineral works synergistically with vitamin E in preventing free radical damage. As part of the antioxidant enzyme glutathione peroxidase, selenium helps maintain a healthy immune system and proper thyroid function. Supplementation appears to boost the immune system by increasing the activity of white blood cells, which attack tumors and microorganisms in the body.

Low levels of selenium have been found in the eyes of those who have cataracts, and increased cancer rates have been reported in areas where there is a low amount of this mineral in the soil. People suffering from rheumatoid arthritis, eczema and psoriasis may also benefit from supplementation with this mineral. Babies who have died from Sudden Infant Death Syndrome (SIDS) have been found to have low levels of selenium in their blood, and SIDS occurs most frequently in those areas of the world with little of this mineral in the soil. The most active forms are selenium-enriched yeast or selenomethionine. Choose these forms over the inorganic salt sodium selenite when supplementing.

Good food sources for selenium include wheat germ, Brazil nuts, oats, red Swiss chard and barley. Recommended daily allowance: 200 mcg.

Sulfur

A constituent of the amino acids cystine, cysteine and methionine, this mineral present in the hair and nails is a vital part of protein metabolism. Though plentiful in foods, sulfur can be very helpful when applied topically to brittle, damaged hair.

Here's how it works: Your hair is made of protein cables tightly wound together.

What keeps the proteins strong are the bonds between the amino acids, which can be attacked and damaged by harsh detergents (such as sodium lauryl sulfate) and other strong chemicals. Sulfur-containing amino acids in shampoos and conditioners can help restore these amino acid bonds and strengthen the hair from the inside out. Herbs such as horsetail and coltsfoot, reputed to be very beneficial to the hair, are high in sulfur.

Exercise and You

According to *Dr. Whitaker's Guide to Natural Healing,* for every hour you exercise, you increase your longevity by two hours. Exercise improves your mood, your energy level, your cardiovascular health and every bodily function. In fact, remaining active is a surefire way to stay young. Whether it's a brisk walk around the block or an hour's jog along the beach, finding an enjoyable activity that raises your heart rate is key to staying healthy. The benefits to your skin are obvious: with increased circulation, the skin cells are better nourished. Perspiration and lipid production are also increased, keeping your skin well-moisturized. With the increased breathing rate that goes with heavy exercise, you take in more oxygen, which in turn increases the production of new cells. Plus added perspiration also helps rid the body of toxins.

Increasingly, research shows that aerobic exercise is not the only way you can stay young by keeping fit. Strength training is also very important, as shown in a ground-breaking study published in the *Journal of the American Medical Association* in 1990. In this study, nursing home residents ranging in age from 86 to 96 lifted weights for eight weeks as part of a supervised program. At the end of two months, these elderly people, most of whom had relied on walkers or canes, had increased their strength an average of 175%. Two participants no longer needed their canes. All found that their walking and balance abilities had improved by an average of 48%.

As women become older, weight gain and osteoporosis are definite concerns, but strength training can prevent and reverse both. As you age, your body loses muscle every year, unless you take steps to reverse this unfortunate process. Strength training builds muscle, which requires more energy to maintain than fat; therefore you burn more calories because your metabolism has been increased. Postmenopausal women lose around one percent of bone mass per year, even more during the first five years after menopause, but according to a Tufts study published in *The Journal of the American Medical Association* in 1994, women who lifted weights gained one percent bone mass during the one-year study. (The control group had lost two percent during the study.) So visit your health club or your local Y and learn more about how to stay young and fit while lifting weights.

Brushing the Skin

Not much has been written about this time-honored skin treatment, but we've found many people who swear by dry-brushing the skin. It's easy to understand why. Dry-brushing with a natural bristle brush or loofah increases circulation, removes dead skin cells and stimulates the skin to optimum levels. Think of it as a workout just for your skin!

Here's how we recommend you do it: Get yourself a good-quality loofah or natural bristle brush, then every day or evening before bathing, gently but firmly brush your skin for five minutes or so. Work the loofah or brush up and down your body and limbs in long strokes. Avoid tender areas, or do these especially gently. You might have to start out easy at first, but keep it up and pretty soon you'll find you can't go without your daily brushing. You'll find it leaves your skin smooth and glowing, and a feeling of well-being all over your body.

IV

The Ingredients

Thirty years ago when Aubrey Organics® began making natural cosmetics, we had to travel all over the world to find certain herbals and other natural ingredients used in our formulas. Many of them were either not available in this country, or were not of sufficient quality to meet our standards. However, due to the incredible growth of the natural products industry over the past decade, it is now possible to go into any health food store and find things you couldn't have found there 10 years ago. Today most natural products retailers will stock a wide variety of high quality herbs, essential oils, supplements and foods—everything you will need to create your own cosmetics at home. You'll even find some of these ingredients at your local drug store or grocery store.

What follows is a comprehensive list of ingredients you will be using, along with some valuable information as to what they are and what they will do for your hair and skin. Read this section carefully and use it as a reference guide as you work with the different formulas. Get to know these ingredients. We've also included some herbs and food supplements that are not used in the formulas *per se*, but that are excellent hair and skin care ingredients and can be added to these formulas or used in other cosmetic recipes that you create yourself.

In the Formulas section we make some recommendations as to specific brands we find to be of high quality, but other brands will do as well. Just remember to read the labels on all ingredients you purchase to make sure they have no synthetic additives or fillers of any kind, and try to buy organic whenever possible. The Resources section of this book will tell you where to call or write if you have difficulty finding any of these ingredients in your local stores.

Acacia (Gum Arabic)

The dried, gummy extract from the stems and branches of *Acacia senegal,* a thorny tree that grows in the Republic of Sudan, which supplies most of the gum arabic to the world. Gum arabic is used in sugar to prevent crystallization, and in other foods as a suspender, emulsifier, stabilizer and flavor fixative. It is also an excellent emulsifying agent for cosmetics, and an important ingredient which provides the "hold" in hairsprays and hair gels, and in natural formulations replaces the less desirable chemical PVP, a type of plastic. (To make a natural hairspray with gum arabic, see Formula #24 in Part V.)

Alcohol (Natural Grain)

This is the pure, natural grain alcohol you can buy right in your neighborhood liquor store. Unlike the petroleum-based synthetic alcohols, it has almost no odor. It is both an excellent disinfectant and a natural preservative, and will help keep your cosmetic formulas stable and free of bacteria, as well as acting as a clearing and purifying agent for your skin. It can be slightly drying, but only if used in too high amounts. If you have trouble obtaining it, a high quality vodka (triple distilled) can be used in its place.

Almond Meal

Almond meal is the ground nut of the almond. A gentle exfoliant, it helps remove dead skin cells that can make your complexion dull and lifeless. Its gentle scrubbing action is not irritating to delicate facial skin, and helps break up oil deposits and debris gently to prevent clogged pores and blemishes. It is a great natural ingredient in masks and scrubs, and you can find it in most health food stores. Just remember to buy organic if you can.

Aloe Vera

There is historical evidence that aloe vera has been used in cosmetic formulations since the time of Cleopatra for its soothing and healing properties. An emollient and skin revitalizer, it remains one of nature's most effective remedies for sunburn and makes an excellent treatment for household burns, cuts and scrapes, and damaged or irritated skin. A hardy plant, aloe grows well in dry soil, and chances are you can grow it at home—either indoors in a large pot, or in your own backyard.

The New Testament mentions aloe as one of the plant extracts used to anoint Christ's body after His death, but the history of the aloe plant goes back much further. The *Papyrus Ebers*, Egyptian texts written around 1500 B.C., are among the oldest documents to record aloe's medicinal powers, and in the first century A.D., Roman naturalist Pliny the Elder wrote extensively on aloe as a healing agent for wounds and skin irritations, and as a tonic for the liver when taken internally. So highly valued was this plant that Aristotle of Stagira (384-322 B.C.), teacher of Alexander the Great, persuaded his imperialistic student to conquer the island of Socotra, in East Africa, just to get their abundant aloe crop to treat soldiers' wounds.

There are two major products derived from the leaves of the aloe: the yellow, bitter juice found beneath the thick epidermis, generally taken internally, and the soft tissue in the center of the leaf that contains a sticky, clear gel, or pulp. Our interest is in the topical use of aloe vera, which involves the pulp, not the juice. Aloe vera gel is 96% water, which makes it an excellent skin and scalp hydrator. Its active ingredients are natural steroids (antiinflammatories), organic acids, enzymes, amino acids, glucomanna and other polysaccharides, as well as chrysophanic acid, an important healing agent to the skin.

Medical studies recently conducted in Egypt have shown that aloe is very beneficial in the treatment of acne, dandruff and seborrhea, and there have been some positive findings related to hair regrowth in seborrheic-related baldness. At the Moscow Stomatological Institute, in Russia, scientific studies have shown that aloe vera extract in water actually regenerated nerve fibers, and some forms of periodontal disease have been successfully treated with aloe vera injections, which were found to influence the activity of cell enzymes in the gums, reducing bleeding and secretion.

An interesting study conducted by I. E. Danhoff, Ph.D., M.D., and B.H. McAnalley, Ph.D., at the Southwest Institute for Natural Resources in Grand Prairie, Texas, used cell cultures from human tissue to observe the effects of aloe vera gel and aloe vera sap on human skin. Scientists found that both the extract of fresh leaves and commercially packaged aloe vera gel had lectin-like substances. Lectins are proteins found primarily in plant seeds that stimulate production of white blood cells, which the body uses to fight disease. Aloe vera's similarity to lectins may be responsible for its wound- and burn-healing properties. The Southwest Institute's research also supports Russian findings concerning the benefits of aloe vera as a healing agent for gum disease.

One of the big problems consumers face when choosing aloe vera-based cosmetics is in the purity of the aloe available. Some methods of extraction involve the use of harsh synthetic chemicals, and the resulting gel products vary considerably. Many commercial, aloe-based cosmetics are so chemicalized that the cellular activity found in the fresh gel is simply not there.

In the Formulas section of this book you will see aloe used quite a bit. We highly recommend you use either certified organic aloe purchased in your health food store, or use the gel from a fresh plant you grow yourself to be certain that chemicals and additives will not compromise the natural action of the aloe. To use the fresh aloe, simply split the leaf, scrape the pulp from the inside, and use as needed.

Amino Acids

Amino acids are the building blocks of protein. There are many types of protein in the body, each with a specific function, each composed of a certain group of amino acids linked together in a specific way. Next to water, these proteins account for the greatest portion of our body weight.

The different proteins that make up the human body are not directly obtained from the diet. Rather, all proteins we eat are broken down into their component amino acids, which are in turn utilized by the body to manufacture the kinds of proteins it needs. Thus, it's the amino acids in proteins, not the proteins themselves, that are the essential nutrients. While most plants and microorganisms are able to use inorganic compounds to manufacture all the amino acids they require, animals (including humans) must obtain some amino acids from their diet.

There are about 28 commonly known amino acids, every one of them important for the growth and maintenance of the body's functions. An amino acid deficiency can lead to serious health problems, including liver damage, anemia and tissue defects. Externally, a deficiency may manifest itself in hair loss, arrested nail growth and a number of skin disorders.

For our purposes, in this book we will focus on the sulfur-containing amino acids—cysteine, cystine and methionine—all essential to protein metabolism. Proper metabolism of sulfur is largely responsible for the healthy condition of our hair and skin.

Of special significance is the evidence that, when applied to the skin and scalp, sulfur-containing amino acids are readily absorbed and utilized by the body to help build healthy keratin, the main protein found in the hair and skin. Results from clinical studies have also shown that cystine and cysteine have a positive effect on seborrhea and other skin and scalp conditions. Methionine is indispensable for growth and skin cell renewal, and as a regulator of lipid metabolism, and is particularly effective in helping control overactive oil glands.

The Natural Almond Amino Acid Shampoo featured in Part V (Formula #17) is intended for application to structurally damaged hair—hair that has become porous, brittle and unmanageable as a result of chronic scalp disorders, invasive hairdressing techniques (dyeing, perms, etc.) or too much exposure to the sun. It is also recommended for scalps with excessive secretion of sebum, leading to very oily hair and dandruff. Amino acid skin creams offer the same oil-regulating properties and are also suitable for very oily skin, combination skin with oily patches, or skin prone to acne and/or blemishes.

By becoming familiar with the different amino acids, you will get to understand their importance to the general health of your body, as well as your hair and skin. Whether taken internally or applied topically, they can make a tremendous difference. The Natural Almond Amino Acid Shampoo mentioned above offers an amino acid blend in an ultra-conditioning formula, and Blue Green Algae Hair Rescue Shampoo (Formula #20) contains an amino acid blend, plus added L-cysteine.

Arnica Oil

Arnica has been a popular and well-proven herbal remedy for centuries. Extracts of arnica blossoms were once an indispensable item in every family's medicine chest, used in poultices and liniments for the treatment of cuts, abrasions and other minor injuries to the skin and tissues. Herbal literature tells us the oil has been successfully used in the treatment of phlebitis, arthritis, bruises, contusions, strained muscles, sprains and slow-healing wounds. Preparations containing arnica are currently used in internal medicine for the oil's ability to strengthen and stimulate the circulatory system. Applied topically, arnica oil has been shown to increase blood flow to the skin, and is used in cosmetics as both a circulation enhancer and an antiinflammatory to help prevent puffiness.

Avocado Oil

Much more than a simple oil base, avocado oil is as an active and nutrient-rich substance very beneficial to the hair and skin because of its special constituents—mainly oleic, linoleic and palmitoleic fatty acids, sterols and vitamins A, D and E.

Its use originated in the tropics, where avocado trees are plentiful. Natives applied the oil directly to the skin to protect it from heat and sun exposure and prevent dryness and chapping. References to its positive effect on dry or flaking skin are found in herbal literature dating back hundreds of years, and this rich oil is often included in preparations for treatment of eczema and other skin disorders.

Avocado oil is useful for its high spreadability. Formulations containing it are easily distributed over the skin for better absorption. It is an excellent addition to cosmetic products that need a natural, "ultra-fine" oil with a protective and softening effect on the skin.

The quality of the oil you buy will vary according to the quality of the fruit from which it was extracted, its ripeness, and the methods used in extraction. Now that avocado oil can be obtained in large quantities due to new production techniques, and in higher quality thanks to better and gentler extraction methods, the cosmetic industry has shown a renewed interest in this excellent emollient.

Barley
(See Green Magma)

Bentonite

Bentonite's name is derived from its place of origin: Benton, Montana. A soft, moisture-absorbing clay mineral, often of volcanic origin, it is often used in exfoliating masks for its drawing and skin-purifying properties. Bentonite can be drying to the skin, so its drying effects must be corrected by adding emollient herbal oils to your clay mixture.

Benzoin Gum

The resin extracted from the bark of various species of an Asian tree, a superb astringent and antiseptic. It is high in antioxidants, and makes an excellent skin protector and natural preservative. Benzoin gum is sometimes used in soaps, face creams, lotions and other cosmetic products, but a synthetic version of it, sodium benzoate, is much more common.

Bilberry Powder

Bilberry is sometimes called the "aviator's herb" because it is of great benefit to the eyes, and has been found to help improve night vision and prevent macular degeneration and other eye problems. Native to Europe, and common throughout much of the British Isles, the bilberry plant bears edible, sweet berries, almost black in color, which have long been a popular food for their high vitamin content.

An astringent and antiseptic, bilberry fruit extract has been used in cosmetic formulations for thousands of years as an ingredient in facial masks and lotions. Its natural fruit acids work gently to tone and rejuvenate the complexion, clear away dead skin cells and debris and help promote skin cell regeneration. (Alpha-hydroxy, the patented trade name for a type of fruit acids, is now found in many commercial skin care products; originally it was used as a solvent in cleaning compounds and in the tanning of leather!) I've used bilberry extract in many exfoliation formulas to smooth and revitalize dull, dry or mature skin. In Part V, our Red Mask Alpha Hydroxy Fruit Acid Treatment (Formula #10) uses bilberry for its exfoliating and skin cell regenerating properties.

Biotin

Sometimes known as vitamin H, biotin is actually a B vitamin. An important factor in healthy tissue growth, it also helps regulate the proper secretion of oils by the sebaceous glands. A biotin deficiency leads to the dry, flaky skin of seborrheic dermatitis, which manifests itself in the formation of dandruff, crusts and gray, sallow skin. Applied topically, biotin is essential for the health of the hair and scalp, and along with PABA (para-aminobenzoic acid) and other B vitamins, is reported to have a beneficial effect in the prevention of hair loss and breakage. (See also Vitamins: B-Complex.) Formula #17, Natural Almond Amino Acid Shampoo, uses biotin as one of its key ingredients.

Black Currant and Borage Oils

In the late 70s and early 80s, evening primrose oil became one of the hottest-selling items in the health food industry, mainly due to its content of gamma-linolenic acid (GLA), an Omega-6 oil reputed to help a long list of ailments, including heart disease, premenstrual syndrome (PMS), eczema, arthritis and even hangovers. (Also see Essential Fatty Acids.) Scientists previously believed GLA could be found in only two sources—mother's milk and evening primrose oil. They were incorrect. Black currant seed oil and borage oil have both been found to contain this important fatty acid, with borage containing the highest concentration of GLA among the three herbal oils.

I have found that for both internal and topical use, borage oil is as good as evening primrose oil, and easier to use for its mild taste and pleasant odor. (Evening primrose oil, by contrast, has an unpleasant smell and strong taste that burns the throat going down.) Besides its high GLA content, borage oil is an excellent antiinflammatory, and a good source of alpha-linoleic acid, another important fatty acid.

Blue Camomile
(See Camomile)

Blue Green Algae
(See Microalgae)

Burdock Root

An antiseptic and antibacterial frequently used in topical preparations for eczema and other skin disorders. Combined with Rosa Mosqueta® oil, it makes an excellent treatment for dry or aging skin.

Calamine

A pink powder made from a natural blend of zinc oxide and a small amount of ferric oxide, calamine is used in lotions, ointments and liniments for the treatment of rashes and other skin reactions. Soothing and healing to the skin, it relieves itching and irritation and reduces inflammation. It is often a key ingredient in preparations for the treatment of poison oak, poison ivy and other less-than-friendly plants. A mixture of calamine and aloe vera makes an excellent skin treatment for burns, rashes and insect bites.

Calendula Oil

Herbalists of the past praise the calendula plant as a remedy for every imaginable injury involving skin or tissue damage. Applied directly to the skin or in the form of poultices and ointments, calendula blossom extracts have been used in the treatment of minor wounds, burns (including sunburn), eczema, abrasions, chapped and chafed skin areas and bedsores with great success. A superb healing agent, calendula oil stimulates the formation of new tissue, helps reduce and prevent inflammation and acts as a mild circulation enhancer.

In herbal cosmetology, its use as a skin toner and soothing agent goes back hundreds of years. Calendula oil is particularly effective in the care of sensitive, easily irritated skin (including a baby's delicate skin), and skin that tends to be dry. It is frequently found in cosmetic formulas for rough, sun-damaged or flaking skin.

Camomile

Camomile has been widely used in cosmetic preparations for thousands of years for its soothing and moisturizing effect on the hair and skin. We use two types of camomile: golden camomile, also known as Roman camomile, which yields a bright yellow oil, and blue camomile, a rare form of the herb whose oil, as the name suggests, is a deep blue.

Golden camomile oil is obtained from the flowers through steam distillation. It has many medicinal properties, including a strong antibacterial and antifungal action (particularly effective against *Candida albicans*), as well as analgesic (pain-relieving), healing and antiinflammatory effects.

Blue camomile contains an oil high in chamazulene, which gives the extract its deep blue color and unique fragrance. Also obtained by steam distillation, blue camomile oil is very expensive and varies considerably, depending on the sources. The highest grade blue camomile oil comes from Morocco.

Extracts of camomile are widely used in cosmetics, including bath elixirs, shampoos, conditioners, sunscreens and mouthwashes. The oils are also used as fragrance components or active ingredients in soaps, detergents, creams, lotions and perfumes. Blue camomile is considered both an excellent deodorant and a stimulant to skin metabolism, while golden camomile oil is often used to bring out highlights in blond hair.

Camomile flowers or extracts are among the most common herbal tea ingredients, either singly or in combination with other herbals, and are used as mild sleep aids, and to relieve stomach disorders (particularly those caused by stress) and poor digestion.

Blue camomile is the key ingredient in my fragrant Blue Camomile Shampoo, formulated over two decades ago, which is still one of our most popular hair products.

Camphor Oil

One of the most overlooked essential oils, camphor is extracted from the gum of the camphor tree, and is excellent in many hair and skin care formulas. Its chief constituent is borneene, a powerful antiseptic. Tiny amounts of the oil are used in aftershave lotions, facial cleansers and cooling skin creams for its freshening and toning properties, and as an antiinflammatory to help combat puffiness. It is a strong oil, so you must use it sparingly, measuring it carefully and adding only a few drops at a time.

Carrot Oil, Carrot Juice

Carrot oil and carrot juice are rich in beta carotene (provitamin A) and tocopherols (vitamin E). Vitamin A (or its provitamin, carotene) is indispensable in maintaining the body's metabolic processes—an imbalance of it can lead to such disorders as night blindness, eye dysfunctions and bone malformations.

A vitamin deficiency (particularly of vitamin A) often makes itself apparent in the skin earlier than in other organs. Thus, the skin can also be regarded as an indicator for an orderly vitamin balance. Vitamin A deficiencies can result in excessively dry skin and premature wrinkles, as well as impaired function of the oil and sweat glands. A lack of vitamin A can also affect hair growth, and may lead to hair loss and some scalp disorders.

Provitamin A is converted into vitamin A in the liver and intestines with the aid of enzymes so that it exerts the same biological actions as vitamin A. For the cosmetic use of provitamin A, it is important that carotene be similarly converted into vitamin A in the sebaceous glands of the skin.

Symptoms of a Vitamin A deficiency manifested in the skin can be treated with topical applications of preparations containing carrot oil. This nutrient-rich oil stimulates the formation of new skin cells, protects the external layers of the skin, helps normalize oil secretion in the skin and scalp and prevents dry, scaly scalp and skin and brittle, lifeless hair.

Castile Soap

Castile soap was originally prepared from olive oil in much the same manner that soap is made from coconut oil. The term is now used to describe a very mild soap; however, the finest grade of castile soap is still made with olive oil. It is often used as a base for natural shampoos and skin cleansers. (In Part V there are several shampoo formulas which have castile as one of their principal ingredients.)

Castor Oil

The history of castor oil (just like Grandma used to give you) spans several millennia and a whole world of geography! The plant is native to India, but also grows easily in Brazil and China, and its seeds yield 25-35% oil, which is remarkably stable and does not turn rancid easily.

In spite of its unpleasant flavor, castor oil is highly regarded as an herbal medicine, particularly as a strong laxative. It is also an excellent healing agent, and mixed into a citron ointment, has been used for centuries in India as a topical treatment for leprosy, skin lesions and abscesses.

Castor oil is high in fatty acids, which makes it extremely beneficial and nourishing to the skin. An excellent lubricant, it is used in lipsticks, hair styling products, creams, lotions and soaps. Because of its high absorption qualities, care should be taken when mixing it with other ingredients, as the oil will cause them to be quickly assimilated into the body.

Cayenne Pepper Oil

In the past two years alone, over 115 clinical studies have been conducted on the effects of cayenne pepper oil on humans. Its active ingredient, *capsaicin*, the chemical responsible for making peppers hot, is also a powerful analgesic and antiinflammatory. Capsaicin works by inhibiting the body's production of substance P, the chemical responsible for the transmission of pain impulses to the central nervous system. Applied topically in the form of ointments and liniments, the effects of cayenne pepper oil are cumulative. It not only prevents the body from producing more substance P, but continued use actually causes the body's reserves of this pain-transmitting chemical to be depleted, thus decreasing our ability to feel pain. Capsaicin has been successfully used to help relieve the symptoms of shingles, neuropathy, arthritis, fibromyalgia and other painful chronic conditions.

In Part V we've included a recipe for a foot massage cream made with cayenne pepper oil, which offers instant relief from soreness and muscle strain and is a Godsend for people who are on their feet a lot. (See Formula #28, Feet Rescue Massage Cream for Troubled Feet.) As you can imagine, cayenne pepper oil is strongly irritating to the eyes, so always wash your hands after handling this "hot" herb, and be sure to keep it away from broken skin or sensitive areas.

Cedarwood Oil

Essential oil frequently used as a fragrance ingredient in soaps, shampoos, creams and perfumes. A known antiirritant, it has a soothing effect on the skin and scalp. (For more information on the use of essential oils, see Fragrances in this section.)

Clay

The use of clay abounds in today's beauty industry. Health food stores usually have a few clay products on their shelves, most (if not all) beauty salons and skin care clinics use it in facial masks, and some European and Japanese spas go as far as to coat the entire body with "healing" clay, burying clients up to their necks in the stuff.

Different regions produce different clays, but the clay most highly prized for cosmetic purposes is kaolin, a white clay that initially could only be obtained from Mt. Kaolin, in China. This mountain supplied the royalty of Europe for generations, and the superb quality of kaolin could not be duplicated in Europe. The Chinese controlled the production of white clay until the expansion of the American frontier brought about the discovery of a western kaolin clay whose high quality could compare with China's.

Kaolin clay mixes easily with water to create a smooth paste or pack that is applied to the skin and allowed to remain on for several minutes. Any clay mask or beauty mask should produce a noticeable tightening effect on the skin, and enough drawing power to pull dirt and debris to the surface and clear and deep-cleanse without irritating the complexion. The tightening and drawing effect is produced when water separates the clay particles, increasing the volume of the clay. As the clay dries through evaporation, the volume decreases, causing the mask to "tighten" on your skin and draw dirt and impurities to the surface.

To make a clay beauty mask, measure out two parts water for every part clay. If the mixture is too dry (after waiting briefly to allow the water to be absorbed by the clay), carefully add more water in small amounts. You may mix honey and other extracts along with the clay to create a massage mask that can be very beneficial to the complexion. Clay tends to be drying, so if you already have a dry complexion, you may want to consider using an herbal mask rather than a clay-based one, or add some moisturizing ingredients into your clay mask. (See Part V for our Green Clay & Blue Green Algae Moisturizing Mask, Formula #7, an excellent, non-drying facial treatment for all skin types.)

Chlorella
(See Microalgae)

Cocoa Butter

Cocoa butter is the solid fat expressed from the seeds of the cocoa plant, used as a lubricant and skin softener in lipsticks, eyelash creams, rouges, soaps and emollient creams. It causes allergic reactions in some people, but if you can tolerate it, cocoa butter is a superb moisturizer and soothing agent. (If you have a sensitivity to cocoa butter, I suggest you substitute it with shea butter, another excellent emollient.)

Coconut Oil

The pure, natural oil obtained from coconuts is an excellent emollient. It can be used to make mild, natural soaps through a saponification reaction with salt. Coconut fatty alcohols and coconut fatty acids are obtained from coconut oil and added to creams, lotions, shampoos and other cosmetics for their soothing and moisturizing properties. But beware: various synthetic chemicals are often added to coconut oil in the making of many cosmetic ingredients, which brings us to our usual advice—read the labels. Often, synthetically processed derivatives of coconut oil, such as sodium lauryl sulfate, are listed in cosmetic labels, followed by the phrase "comes from coconuts." This is misleading. Remember: if it's too long to pronounce, it's probably synthetic. Accept nothing but the real thing in its natural form.

Cod Liver Oil

The pale yellow fatty oil extracted from the fresh livers of some species of codfish is extremely high in vitamins A and D. Just one gram of cod liver oil contains about 400,000 I.U. of vitamin A and about 40,000 I.U. of vitamin D-3. A respected therapeutic agent for more than a century, cod liver oil was first used as a vitamin D supplement for children, an important nutrient often missing from their diets. It was introduced into dermatology later as a topical treatment. Since then there have been a large number of preparations formulated with cod liver oil, and the literature on the subject is probably more extensive than on any other topical ingredient. Cod liver oil is employed mainly to promote the healing of wounds and in the treatment of skin damage and inflammation.

Attempts to incorporate the oil into cosmetic preparations have been thwarted by its characteristic, unpleasant odor, which cannot be masked even by strong perfumes. As a result, concentrates containing cod liver oil's active ingredients in high proportions have been developed. These concentrates still have a strong odor, but can be used in much smaller amounts, minimizing the problem.

Cod liver oil is ideal for very sensitive skin (especially a baby's skin) and for rough, chapped, cracked or irritated skin. It is an excellent treatment for "dishpan hands" and chapped or sun-damaged skin.

Cold Cream

Cold cream is possibly the world's first commercially sold cosmetic product. It was developed around 150 A.D. by the Greek physician Galen, who combined almond oil and beeswax into a water and rosewater base, and put his slaves to work 'round the clock creating small batches of the cream. This rich cream was in great demand, but was unstable and spoiled quickly.

Cosmetic manufacturers who came after Galen discovered that by adding about 0.5% borax, a whiter-looking, more stable cream could be made. Much later on, various chemicals such as petrolatum, Tween 40, mineral oil, glyceryl monostearate, ozokerite, methyl and propyl paraben and other synthetics made their way into Galen's original formula, and the cosmetic face cream found in most drugstores today was born.

In the Formulas section you will learn to make your own tofu-based natural cold cream, which is used as an absorption base in many of the cosmetics you'll be creating here. (See Formula #1, Natural Absorption Base, in Part V.) (See also Essential Fatty Acids in this section.)

Collagen

This dermal protein makes up 70% of the body's connective tissue, and gerontologists have found this is where the aging process of the skin takes place. Young connective tissue is made up of flexible, or "soluble" collagen. As the skin ages and is exposed to sunlight, environmental pollutants and chemicals (such as synthetic cosmetic products), the soluble collagen begins to deteriorate and become inflexible, losing its elasticity and its ability to absorb moisture. As a result, the connective tissue becomes tight and dry, causing the skin to wrinkle and age.

Extensive tests by both European and American researchers have shown that soluble collagen, when applied topically, is readily absorbed by the skin and helps slow down collagen loss and replenish moisture and elasticity. However, the skin can only utilize a collagen that is structurally intact. Certain petrochemicals (particularly synthetic preservatives, such as methyl and propyl paraben) found in many collagen-based creams can react with the collagen and make it insoluble and unusable by the skin. We use only pure, soluble collagen from bovine sources in our natural formulas.

Coltsfoot
(See Horsetail, Coltsfoot and Nettle)

Comfrey

A known antiinflammatory, comfrey is very beneficial in skin care products for its healing and moisturizing action. Allantoin, an extract of comfrey root, is used in celltherapy creams for its high content of mucopolysaccharides, substances that bind with water to form the thick, jelly-like material that cements cells together. (Comfrey is not recommended for internal use without a doctor's supervision, as too large a dose may cause liver damage.)

Coneflower

High in fatty acids and plant sterols, coneflower is used in creams and lotions to improve texture and help firm the skin. It is a good addition to anti-wrinkle creams and celltherapy treatments, particularly when combined with aristolochia and aloe.

Part IV — The Ingredients

Corn Meal
The meal obtained from ground corn, used as a thickener and mild exfoliant in cosmetic formulations. It has a soothing and softening effect on the skin.

Cypress Oil
Essential oil frequently used in aromatherapy treatments. (Also see Fragrances.)

Elder Berries
A mild astringent. Its essential oil is high in fatty acids (66%), and very beneficial to the hair and skin.

Essential Fatty Acids (EFA's)
The polyunsaturated fatty acids were recognized about 50 years ago as being vital to the organism. Sometimes known as vitamin F, two types are considered "essential" fatty acids because they cannot be manufactured by the body and must be obtained from the diet—linoleic acid (Omega-6) and linolenic acid (Omega-3). Flaxseed, evening primrose and Rosa Mosqueta® oils, used in many of the formulas in this book, are excellent sources of essential fatty acids, or EFA's.

A deficiency of EFA's results in such disorders as arrested growth, kidney and liver damage, anemia, and susceptibility to infections. This deficiency also manifests itself externally as dry, flaking or sallow skin, generally poor condition of the hair and scalp, and even hair loss. EFA's are used by the body in the production of sebum, your skin's own natural oil, so including these substances in skin products makes good sense. Numerous clinical studies have also shown that EFA's inhibit the growth of bacteria and help raise the body's ability to fight infection, thus they are often included in ointments for skin infections, burns and wounds, as well as in preparations for the treatment of eczema and other skin conditions. Cosmetically, EFA's are recommended for topical application to rough, dry or mature skin and weak or brittle nails, as well as in conditioning treatments for dull, damaged hair and problem scalp.

Eucalyptus Oil
A superb disinfectant and skin purifier, this fragrant essential oil is used in facial cleansers, soaps and bath products for its strong antimicrobial properties. It was introduced into France from Australia in the 1850s, and eucalyptus trees were soon planted in fever-stricken districts of Algiers and Sicily, where their aromatic leaves acted as air cleansers and the drying action of their roots on marshy soils helped prevent the spread of disease-carrying mosquitoes.

Perhaps the most powerful antiseptic of its class, this richly scented oil is an excellent analgesic and antiinflammatory. A natural expectorant, it can relieve sinus and bronchial swelling and congestion and help soothe a sore throat. Its cooling and soothing effect on the skin also makes it an ideal ingredient for massage lotions and ointments for sore muscles. In Part V you will find several formulas that use eucalyptus oil.

Evening Primrose Oil
For centuries Native American healers have used parts of the evening primrose

in poultices to heal wounds and in teas to treat asthma and upset stomachs. Today researchers believe the oil extracted from the evening primrose possesses a dazzling range of health benefits, from relieving the symptoms of premenstrual syndrome (PMS) to clearing up eczema. Scientists are even exploring the oil's potential as a treatment for heart disease, diabetes, chronic fatigue syndrome, arthritis and even alcoholism. All and all, evening primrose oil sounds like a medicine show snake oil, but research indicates it could make a real difference in some people's lives.

Its strong healing powers are attributed to high concentrations of essential fatty acids, particularly gamma-linolenic acid (GLA), which is also found in black currant and borage oils. (High levels of GLA are also present in human breast milk, and some scientists speculate that it may help stimulate brain development in babies.)

Current research indicates that sufferers from atopic eczema show a block in their body's production of GLA. Consequently, a growing number of dermatologists in Europe now recommend taking evening primrose oil for two to three months to help alleviate skin problems associated with eczema and other skin disorders. Primrose oil creams and lotions are very effective in many cases, and many sufferers report improved skin texture and substantial relief from itching and irritation.

The topical use of evening primrose oil on the hair and scalp has also shown promising results. In shampoos, conditioners and rinses, it has a moisturizing effect on dry hair and flaky scalp, and like jojoba oil, it helps regulate oil production, reducing excessive flow of oils without drying out the hair.

Some sources report success using primrose oil for the treatment of psoriasis, but these are not scientific studies. Here is how the oil was used on psoriasis sufferers: 10 to 15 minutes before a shower, the subjects applied pure primrose oil directly onto the lesions, which resulted in intense itching, but caused the hard scales to soften. The subjects then carefully washed all the oil off (which reduced the itching somewhat), then used a rough towel to "massage" the scales. They finished by applying a body lotion containing evening primrose oil directly on the lesions. This method seemed to loosen hard scales, which in turn allowed for a more effective treatment of the lesions. Used on a daily basis, the oil increasingly reduced the itching to the point where there was no more itching when applied.

There is still not enough proof as to whether this is a good long term treatment for the disease, but it appears to be beneficial on a short term basis, as it causes the heavy scales to soften and break off. The main problem in treating psoriasis with evening primrose oil is its strong, unpleasant smell. (It also may leave a ring in the bathtub if not thoroughly washed afterwards, but these difficulties are minor.) A more scientific medical study of evening primrose's effect on psoriasis might prove very interesting.

By combining evening primrose oil with other essential fatty acids in a natural cream base, you can create a light, natural moisturizer for the complexion and the body. This cream is excellent for relieving the inflammation, redness and itching of eczema, and can be used as a baby lotion to help fight and prevent diaper rash. (See Formula #16, Evening Primrose Hand & Body Lotion.)

Fennel

An antibacterial, fennel has a slight tightening and firming action on the skin, which makes it an excellent addition to skin tonics, masks and lotions. It is rich in oleic and linoleic acids, essential fatty acids very beneficial to the skin.

Flaxseed Oil, Flaxseed Meal

In the supplements section of this book (Part III), you read extensively about the importance of flaxseeds and flaxseed oil to your body, particularly the skin. Flaxseeds are rich in Omega-3 essential fatty acids, B-vitamins, protein and minerals. They have a pleasant, nutty taste and can be ground and eaten in salads, soups, cereals and baked goods. Or you may opt to buy the cold-pressed oil and take it straight or use it as a salad oil. (Heating the oil, however, breaks down the natural essential fatty acids, so it should not be used as a cooking oil.)

Studies have shown flaxseed oil can relieve the pain and inflammation of arthritis, and has been found to lower blood cholesterol and triglyceride levels. A tablespoon of flaxseed oil once a day will also, in many cases, get rid of dry skin. In cosmetics both flaxseed oil and flaxseed meal have a positive effect on the skin and hair.

Fragrances

If you opened a jar of complexion cream and discovered it smelled exactly like a bottle of vitamins, you probably wouldn't relish the thought of putting it on your face. In the past we have compounded many natural cosmetics that did not smell too pretty. I believed in using certain natural ingredients for their beneficial effects on the hair and skin, not for the attractiveness of their fragrance. However, in time I learned that by blending certain essential oils into the formula, we could create a more pleasant experience for the user of the product. But more importantly, I discovered essential oils have powerful therapeutic effects, both when inhaled and when absorbed through the skin. (Most essential oils have fantastic absorption capabilities.) One example of an essential oil that delivers not only a calming, delightful fragrance, but also has a toning and moisturizing effect on the hair and skin is blue camomile oil, one of the most exotic and expensive aromatic oils around.

Essential oils are naturally extracted from herbs, or from the roots and bark of plants through steam distillation or cold pressing, and can be applied topically (either straight or blended with water or vegetable oils) in washes, creams and massage lotions, or as inhalants in aromatherapy treatments. In aromatherapy, aromatic essential oils are utilized as active ingredients to stimulate the natural healing action of both the body and the mind. When you have a cold or a clogged nose and use a medicated inhaler to draw the vapors into your nasal passages, this is a modern application of aromatherapy. The old herbal remedy of a chest rub is another form of aromatherapy at work.

The use of aromatic oils dates back more than 5,000 years, to the ancient Egyptians, who used them medicinally and in religious ceremonies, as well as in beauty products and perfumes. The healing and restorative properties of these oils were well known to ancient practitioners, but became all but forgotten for generations.

Many people believe they are allergic to essential oils, and it's easy to understand why, since it is the fragrance component of a cosmetic that causes the most allergic reactions. More than likely, though, it is the synthetic fragrances added to most cosmetic preparations, not the natural fragrance oils, that are causing the problem. Most fragrances used today are complex mixtures of synthetic chemicals that are as far from a flower as a smokestack is from a green meadow. Practically every commercial cosmetic product—from the most inexpensive shampoo to the finest French perfume—contains synthetic fragrance oils. Even so-called "fragrance-free" products use fragrance ingredients to mask the smell of the other ingredients, thus giving the product its "no-scent" aroma. Since FDA labeling laws do not require the specific listing of fragrance in a product, masking ingredients in "fragrance-free" formulas will not be listed on the label.

In the mainstream cosmetic industry, fragrance belongs to the merchandising area, not to the chemist. Like color and packaging, it is a point-of-purchase consideration. Many cosmetic manufacturers believe the look and smell of a product are the keys to its success or failure in the marketplace, and a great deal of time and money is spent trying to determine which fragrances will sell the best. A product's scent is designed to enhance the consumer's perception of the product, thus a cream or lotion marketed as a beauty product must smell "beautiful," while a medicated product will have a strong medicinal smell, so you know it's working. These fragrances usually have little to do with the active ingredients; they are there to make the product smell good enough to sell. Thus, a commercial avocado face cream is colored a vivid green with FD & C Yellow #5 and FD & C Blue #2, and scented with a synthetic mixture created in the lab to smell like avocados. The eyes and nose tell us this is avocado cream, but alas there is little avocado oil in it. (Avocado oil, incidentally, is amber-colored and practically odorless.)

You will be using many essential oils—both for their therapeutic effects and their natural fragrances—in your cosmetic formulas, so it's important to get acquainted with the different oils available. Today skin care clinics use essential oils during aromatherapy relaxation techniques, but they are also an important component in facial treatments because they facilitate cellular nutrition and promote skin cell renewal. There are also aromatherapy treatments to encourage hair growth and revitalize dull, lackluster or thinning hair and problem scalp.

An excellent source of information on aromatherapy and the proper use of many essential oils is Robert B. Tisserand's *The Art of Aromatherapy* (Inner Traditions International, 1977). When purchasing essential oils, it's important to read the label and make sure no synthetic chemicals have been added, and that the base for the oils is natural (i.e., jojoba, peanut, sunflower oils, etc.).

Ginger

Available as both a powder and an oil, ginger is a stimulant and antiirritant, as well as a strong antimicrobial and antioxidant. Used topically, it promotes circulation and helps reduce inflammation, and its warming and soothing properties are very beneficial to the skin. Sometimes used in commercial formulations as a fragrance, ginger's therapeutic properties have been completely overlooked by the cosmetic industry, but not by me. I've been using ginger in my formulas since 1967, when I included powdered ginger in Relax-R-Bath, the first Aubrey Organics® product. (See Formula #26, Kava Kava Relaxing Bath Emulsion, a "Relax-R-Bath" you can make right at home.)

Grain Alcohol
(See Alcohol, Natural Grain)

Grapefruit Seed Extract

The bitter extract from grapefruit seeds is a powerful antimicrobial and antifungal, and an excellent natural preservative. Early on, Aubrey Organics® products were preserved with a blend of antioxidant vitamins (A, C and E). In the early 70s, Dr. Jakob Harich approached us with a remarkable discovery. Dr. Steven Otwell and Dr. Wayne Marshall, leading researchers on the effects of microbes on food at the University of Florida, in Gainesville, were among the first scientists to corroborate Dr. Harich's findings, which established grapefruit seed extract had an astonishing capacity to protect fruits, vegetables, poultry and fish from the assault of bacteria, fungi and parasites.

The next area Dr. Harich wanted to explore was the extract's ability to preserve cosmetic formulations, and I began a series of tests to determine the effectiveness of grapefruit seed extract in cosmetic products. Grapefruit seed extract's antibacterial and antifungal properties proved excellent in protecting the products from bacteria and fungi and keeping them stable for up to a year (and sometimes longer). I combined it with my antioxidant vitamin blend, and with neem oil, another powerful antifungal, and Aubrey Organics® signature natural preservative was born.

In the early 90s, holistic health practitioners in the U.S. began to recommend grapefruit seed extract to people suffering from systemic yeast infections and other fungus-related disorders, and the Pasteur Institute of France, Europe's leading AIDS research center, has been studying the extract's potential as a treatment for both the HIV virus and some secondary infections associated with AIDS. Some European farmers add a powdered form of the extract to animal feed to help ward off the spread of salmonella and E. coli, two potentially lethal bacteria.

As a broad spectrum antimicrobial, grapefruit seed extract has no known toxicity and causes virtually no allergic reactions in most people, and many individuals sensitive to antifungal drugs are better able to tolerate it. Ten drops of the extract in a glass of juice (remember, it is bitter!) three times a day has been shown to turn around the problem of candidiasis. (The extract is also available in capsules; one 125 ml. capsule twice daily should do the job.)

Grapefruit seed extract is both gentler and more effective than the most common disinfectant used in hospitals, isopropyl alcohol, a harsh synthetic that's very drying to the skin. We include it in a number of the formulas in this book, not only as a natural preservative, but also as an active ingredient in acne preparations. Acne occurs when the skin is unable to mount a proper defense against microbes (which is why many dermatologists prescribe antibiotics to help control breakouts). We have found that no more than five drops of grapefruit seed extract added to a facial cleanser or liquid soap will get rid of acne-causing bacteria and should help clear up your complexion within a couple of weeks.

Grapefruit seed extract is also an effective topical treatment against athlete's foot, nail fungi, cold sores, diaper rash and contact dermatitis.

Green Kamut®

Green Kamut® is a registered trademark of Kamut International, Ltd. To make it, kamut, one of the most nourishing foods around, and alfalfa, another superb nutrient, are planted together on high altitude organic farmland, where seasonal run-off from the surrounding volcanic mountains assures maximum nutrition in each harvest. The leaves are harvested, rinsed, juiced and dried within minutes at only 88 degrees, yielding a completely non-pasteurized product. The high protein and mineral content of Green Kamut® makes it an excellent ingredient for a skin-nourishing beauty mask. (Formula #7, Green Clay & Blue Green Algae Moisturizing Mask, uses Green Kamut®.)

Green Magma®

A trademark of Green Foods Corp., Green Magma® is a powdered form of the juice from young barley leaves, grown organically in Japan. Very high in nutrients, including chlorophyll, flavonoids and all the essential amino acids, barley is an excellent antiinflammatory and helps promote digestion. Green Magma® contains thousands of enzymes to aid metabolism and encourage proper assimilation. It is an excellent skin nutrient.

Green Tea

Both a gentle stimulant and a soothing drink, and second only to water in worldwide popularity, green tea was discovered in China over 4,000 years ago when the leaves of a species of white camellia were steeped in hot water and drunk. Green tea was touted as a great tonic and healer as far back as 729 A.D., when Japanese monks began growing the shrubs for use in their religious rituals.

Today powdered *Matcha* green tea remains the beverage of choice for Japan's sacred tea ceremony, an agent of spiritual healing and centering, but its medicinal properties are becoming more and more widely accepted in the West as scientific evidence of its health benefits continues to grow.

The main difference between green tea and the black tea more commonly drunk in Europe and America is in the roasting and preparation of the leaves. Green tea leaves are prepared in a simpler way: the leaves are steamed, rolled and dried, and (unlike black tea) are not fermented. One of the vital ingredients found in green tea, *Epigallocatechin gallate*, is lost during fermentation, thus the unfermented green tea is believed to have more healthful properties.

The popularity of green tea throughout the health food industry has grown by leaps and bounds. Findings of the last 15 years indicate that a few cups of green tea daily may help the body fight off some forms of cancer, reduce the risk of heart disease, strengthen the immune system and even play a role in preventing tooth decay.

But what can it do for your hair and skin? Topically applied, polyphenols in green tea (particularly the previously mentioned *Epigallocatechin gallate*, an antioxidant 20 times stronger than vitamin E) have been proven to help keep tissues healthy by protecting cells from free radical damage caused by environmental pollutants and sun exposure.

Green tea actually functions as an antimutagen—that is, it prevents healthy cells from mutating into cancerous ones. Recent studies conducted by Laboratory for Cancer Research at Rutgers University concluded that green tea polyphenols appeared to inhibit the growth of some skin cancers caused by the sun's UV rays, while similar studies in Japan indicated a decrease in the incidence of skin cancer among people who drank as little as one cup of green tea daily. As a suncare ingredient, green tea is also known to increase the effectiveness of sunscreens (PABA, titanium dioxide and herbal sunblocks) to protect the skin from UV ray damage.

Xanthines found in green tea (theobromine, theophylline and caffeine) have also been shown to help reduce skin irritation and swelling. Known for their strong anti-inflammatory properties, they act as soothing agents to help lessen allergic reactions and relieve the itching and flaking of many skin and scalp conditions. Xanthines, particularly theophylline, are also reputed to help combat the appearance of cellulite, which makes green tea an excellent ingredient in massage creams and anticellulite formulas.

Gum Arabic
(See Acacia.)

Henna

Of the many cosmetic ingredients whose discovery and use are attributed to Cleopatra, henna is the one most commonly associated with her, yet the use of henna definitely predates her by more than a thousand years. It is often thought of as a hair color, but was also used to dye the nails, the palms and soles of the feet of dancers, and the manes and tails of horses. Still, many people don't know henna is also a superb hair conditioning ingredient.

Although it works well on all hair types, it is most effective on oily hair or dry-to-normal hair that has a tendency to become oilier as the day progresses. It also helps loosen scalp buildup and prevent flaking and irritation. The coloring ingredient (lawsone) can be removed from the henna so that it will condition your hair without adding color.

A henna shampoo that will bring out warm highlights in dark hair can be made by mixing 5% henna extract and 5% boric acid in a shampoo base. You can make this up fresh in your kitchen, but be sure to wear rubber gloves, as the henna may stain your fingers.

The main asset to henna as a coloring agent is that it is practically the only widely available, semipermanent hair color that is nontoxic and is not likely to irritate the skin or scalp. (Several henna-based coloring preparations should be available at your health food store.) One disadvantage is that henna does not always color predictably. If you want satisfactory results, you must read the directions on the package carefully and follow them exactly. Fair or gray-haired people in particular need to try out the henna color on a few strands before applying it all over the hair.

People who are using temporary hair rinses should not use henna colorings, as the different coloring agents may mix unfavorably to create a surprising "Technicolor" effect. People with perms should also avoid it, as the henna may interfere with the waving process, or may "take" differently on permed hair.

Herbal Liquid Body Soap

Natural liquid soap available from Aubrey Organics®, used as an ingredient in some recipes for shampoos, cleansers and bath products. This mild formula features a long list of skin-conditioning herbals in a rich almond protein, coconut oil and castile soap base. You can use another natural liquid soap in its place, but you'd be hard pressed to find a gentler and more skin-friendly formula.

Horse Chestnut

One of the main benefits of horse chestnut extract lies in its ability to stimulate blood flow and promote circulation to areas poorly supplied with blood. High in B vitamins, flavonoids and amino acids, horse chestnut extracts, notably aescin, also possess antiinflammatory properties and help prevent fluid retention.

Extracts of horse chestnut fruits, bark and/or seeds have been used for years in the topical treatment of many skin disorders, in creams and lotions for sensitive or irritated skin, and in products to help combat cellulitis. Leaf preparations are used in European folk medicine for eczema, varicose veins, phlebitis and to reduce swelling caused by sprains or bone fractures.

It is well documented that individual vitamins have a greater effect when in the company of other vitamins than when they are applied separately, and combining them with certain herbal extracts or essential oils can bring about a synergistic action—that is, their effectiveness can be increased many times over. The combination of horse chestnut extract and certain vitamins is particularly recommended for skin with over or underactive sebaceous glands—that is, both for dry, rough, scaly skin and for skin with a tendency to greasiness, as well as skin poorly supplied with blood.

Horse chestnut extract has been widely used in shampoos, shower gels and other bath products, as well as complexion care formulas, body and hand creams and lotions, and toothpastes. Cosmetic use in Europe has been based on its antiirritant and skin-clearing properties.

Horsetail, Coltsfoot and Nettle

Folk medicine holds certain plants to be particularly beneficial to the hair, and none are held in as high esteem as horsetail, coltsfoot and nettle, sometimes referred to as the "hair care trio."

Very high in sulfur, silicic acid and amino acids (cystine in particular), horsetail and coltsfoot have long been used in the treatment of various hair disorders such as dandruff, scalp buildup and hair loss. According to recent biochemical literature, scalps with a strong growth of hair have a higher content of silicic acid than scalps with thinning hair. Horsetail is one of the most silica-rich plants around, and its topical use has been shown to help strengthen the hair and promote growth. Coltsfoot has been praised by herbalists for centuries as a superb treatment for problem skin and scalp, and herbal literature contains recommendations for the use of this herb in regulating overactive oil glands.

An excellent hair tonic, nettle extract has also been used in hair care formulas for generations for its high silica and sulfur content. In addition, herbal literature emphasizes nettle's ability to promote circulation to scalps poorly supplied with blood, and to stimulate hair growth when applied directly to the scalp.

I often combine this herbal "hair care trio" with B vitamins, particularly d-panthenol, a hair thickener and natural hydrator, and inositol, essential for cell respiration. Applied topically, B vitamins help regulate excess oil production, and have proven beneficial in the treatment of seborrheic dermatitis and other skin and scalp conditions.

Jojoba Oil

The jojoba (pronounced ho-ho-ba) desert plant hails from North America (Mexico and parts of the U.S. in particular), where it manages to thrive in a hostile environment with a surprising average life span of over 100 years. Few plants could withstand desert temperatures reaching up to 115° F, sparse rainfall and poor soil conditions. Jojoba, however, has a built-in survival mechanism. During the summer months, when the rain almost never falls, the pores of the plant (stomata) are completely sealed by a waxy substance that dramatically reduces the rate of evaporation to help keep moisture in. This wax is concentrated in the beans of the jojoba plant, which are harvested in quantities of up to twelve pounds per plant.

I began working with jojoba oil in my labs in 1972. I was so impressed with this remarkable plant that I created a shampoo and conditioner, and began selling the pure extract as a complexion oil. I also formulated a deep-cleansing facial mask from the jojoba meal left over after the oil has been extracted from the beans. Its increasing popularity as a cosmetic ingredient led many manufacturers to add products containing jojoba oil to their lines, and one company (Wickhen Products, Inc.) actually created an artificial jojoba oil. The formula section of this book contains a number of recipes using real jojoba oil, not a synthetic copy. As you might imagine, jojoba oil is a hard-working hair and skin moisturizer that helps make "desert-dry" hair and skin soft and supple. (Plus it helps control dandruff by keeping the scalp healthy.)

Kava Kava

The use of kava kava originated in the South Pacific, where a drink made from the plant's roots was given to tribal elders for its soothing, centering effect and as an aid in meditation. Much has been written about its usefulness as a sleep aid and its calming properties on the mind. However, many people are not aware of kava kava's effects on the body, as both a pain reliever and muscle relaxant. Widely known in Europe since the 1850s, kava kava's medicinal properties run the gamut. Taken internally, it has been used in the treatment of epilepsy, rheumatism, gout, urinary tract infections, bronchitis, toothaches, headaches and muscle cramps. I have found that a bath emulsion containing this soothing herb works fast to help ease muscle soreness and tension, relieve arthritis pain and help relax both body and mind.

Lavender Oil

This aromatic essential oil is most widely known as a fragrance ingredient, but we use it in creams, lotions and facial astringents for its skin-toning properties, and as a mild antiseptic and soothing agent. A gentle sedative, lavender oil is frequently used in aromatherapy to help combat stress and mild depression.

L-Cysteine

A sulfur-containing amino acid present in the hair protein keratin, cysteine is said to help repair and rebuild damaged, overprocessed hair and have a beneficial effect on the skin and scalp. It is found in many hair care products either as part of an amino acid complex, or as a component in horsetail and coltsfoot, herbals high in this hair-nourishing amino acid. Shampoos and conditioners which contain both herbs are excellent "hair savers." (See also Amino Acids.)

Lecithin

Lecithin is an important constituent of living cells. Cell membranes, which regulate the passage of nutrients in and out of the cell, are largely made up of lecithin. It is composed primarily of the B vitamins choline and inositol, and linoleic acid, and is naturally available in many foods, especially egg yolks and unrefined, cold-pressed vegetable oils. Taken internally, lecithin helps the body digest and disperse fats, protecting the vital organs and arteries from fatty buildup, and also helps improve absorption of fat-soluble vitamins.

In cosmetic formulations, lecithin is often used as an emulsifier and carrying agent, as an emollient for dry hair and skin, and to help offset the drying effects of certain ingredients (particularly synthetic detergents and other chemicals found in mass produced cosmetics).

Of the types of lecithin available, soya lecithin is the most widely used. Since it does not readily mix with water, incorporating soya lecithin into water-based cosmetic preparations can be challenging. In the formula section we will show you how to prepare it so it will be quickly dispersed without clumping.

Lemon Blossom Body Splash

Light splash-on cologne made from herbs and plant essences. An Aubrey Organics® natural product. (For more information on the use of essential oils, see Fragrances in this section.)

Lemon Peel Oil

Native to Asia, the lemon tree is cultivated worldwide, especially in the U.S. (California and Florida). Lemon oil is usually extracted from the peel by cold expression, while petitgrain oil is obtained from the leaves, twigs and undeveloped fruits through steam distillation.

Much milder than lemon juice, lemon oil is composed mainly of limonene (70%), and is commonly used as a flavoring agent, and in very small amounts (less than 1%) as a fragrance in soaps, lotions, creams and colognes. It has mild astringent properties and is a superb skin freshener. Even gentler on the skin, lemon petitgrain oil has been reported to be nonirritating, nonsensitizing and antiinflammatory.

Licorice Root

Licorice root is native to Eurasia, and cultivated in parts of Europe, the Middle East and China. Often used as a flavoring agent, it is known to exhibit strong medicinal traits, including antiinflammatory, antiallergic and antitoxic properties.

Licorice extract has been successfully used in China in the clinical treatment of many illnesses, including gastric and duodenal ulcers, bronchial asthma and contact dermatitis, and flavonoids in licorice root have recently been shown to have strong antioxidant properties. An important element in licorice, known as glabridin, has been shown to delay the oxidation of LDL, the main contributing factor to increased cholesterol on the arterial walls. (Licorice candy does not contain glabridin and therefore has no cholesterol-lowering ability.)

In cosmetics, licorice root has a soothing and detoxifying effect on the skin and scalp and helps ward off allergic reactions and reduce puffiness.

Microalgae
(Chlorella, Spirulina and Blue Green Algae)

Imagine, if you can, a perfect food that has the power to stimulate the immune system, improve digestion, detoxify the body, enhance growth and tissue repair, accelerate healing, protect against ultraviolet radiation and environmental pollutants, help prevent degenerative disease and promote longevity, and that also contains lots of high quality protein, fiber and many of the benefits of leafy greens.

Now imagine not one, but three of these perfect nutrients. What are these marvelous foods and what will they do for the hair and skin, as well as for the body? Blue green algae, spirulina and chlorella are now sold in powder, tablet or supplement fruit drink forms. Let's look at these superb nutrients more closely.

– Chlorella –

Widely known for its disease-fighting properties, this amazing micronutrient is also said to help slow down the aging process. A single-celled organism, chlorella is used widely in Japan, where it has been recognized for 40 years as one of nature's most perfect foods. Grown in clear, clean water, this therapeutic green algae has more RNA (ribonucleic acid) and chlorophyll than any other food source (five to 10 times more chlorophyll than spirulina, and 10 times the amount in alfalfa). Chlorophyll is recognized for its ability to speed the cleansing of the bloodstream, and RNA, a major ingredient in new blood cells, helps protect tissues against the effects of ultraviolet rays and pollution.

Chlorella is made up of 60% protein, and is high in vitamins A, B-2, B-6, B-12, C, K and E, as well as some important minerals and antioxidants, including calcium, magnesium, iron, zinc, phosphorus, iodine and beta carotene. In addition, chlorella contains 19 of the 28 essential and nonessential amino acids.

Chlorella also makes an excellent topical treatment. Because of its superb healing properties, this wonder powder can be used for cleansing the complexion, and as a soothing wash for damaged or irritated skin. Combined with aloe vera, it makes a perfect acne treatment that helps clear up breakouts and blemishes and leaves the skin fresh and smooth.

You will be using chlorella in some of your natural recipes. But remember, you will also have it on hand to take internally as a nutrient. Here are some of the other claims made for chlorella: Taken regularly, it detoxifies the body of pollutants, prevents constipation, promotes bowel health and helps fight off infection. Peptic and duodenal ulcers, symptoms of high stress living, respond well to chlorella supplementation, particularly when used in conjunction with prescribed medications. Chlorella is also high in beta carotene and vitamin E, powerful antioxidants that actually work together to prevent cancer. Recommended daily dosage is one to three tsp. of powder mixed into juice or water. (Amount depends on your age, weight and needs.)

– Spirulina –
According to Helen C. Morgan and Kelly J. Moorhead (*Spirulina: Nature's Superfood*), this microalgae grew wild for thousands of years in the great lakes of Central Mexico, where it was prized by the Aztecs as a food source.

Robert Henrikson, president of Earthrise Co. (which produces Earthrise spirulina), documents in *The Ultimate Guide to Health & Fitness* that spirulina is currently being used in Third World countries to treat malnutrition. Malnourished infants taking three to 15 grams of spirulina a day show rapid weight gain. In China, Nanjing Children's Hospital uses it regularly in some baby formulas to help infants recover from a variety of nutritional deficiencies. Its high protein level, easy digestibility and concentration of vitamins, minerals and essential fatty acids make it ideal for therapeutic and nutritional use.

According to Henrikson, spirulina has a higher concentration of protein (60%), amino acids, beta carotene, vitamin B-12, gamma-linolenic acid and trace minerals than any other natural food source. It is also the only natural food containing all the essential and nonessential amino acids

– Blue Green Algae –
Blue green algae, the most primitive of these microalgae, is also very commonly used as a nutrient. It differs from spirulina and chlorella in that its cell wall is made from glycogen and is very easily digested. One of nature's earliest food sources, blue green algae is composed of 50 to 71% protein, all the major amino acids, plus 12-15% minerals and trace minerals and a long list of vitamins. Its high glycogen content makes it excellent for cell growth and especially beneficial to the hair and scalp.

Both blue green algae and spirulina contain phycocyanin, a blue-green pigment that may help prevent some cancers. A Japanese patent application states that daily ingestion of a small dosage of phycocyanin accelerates normal cell growth and inhibits the growth of malignant tumors in cancer patients. In 1989 *The Journal of the National Cancer Institute* (Volume 16) stated that glycolipids extracted from blue green algae have been found to inhibit the AIDS virus in experimental studies.

Later on you will learn how to formulate a blue green algae hair mask that will help clear up scalp problems and relieve the bothersome symptoms of psoriasis, seborrhea and other disorders. This pre-shampoo conditioning treatment softens and moisturizes the hair and adds body and shine, and will actually help stop hair from falling out!

Milk Thistle
In recent years, few herbal extracts have been as extensively studied as milk thistle. Milk thistle seeds were first mentioned as a treatment for liver conditions by Roman naturalist Pliny the Elder in the 1st century A.D. High in antioxidants (10

times higher than vitamin E), milk thistle's ability to reduce toxic reactions indeed make it an excellent liver protector. Clinical studies suggest that it inhibits liver damage caused by alcohol abuse and exposure to industrial chemicals, protects against the absorption of toxins, and stimulates the normal function of the liver.

Milk thistle extract used in facial and body lotions and moisturizers has a soothing and calming effect on the skin. Applied topically, it's valuable for the skin for its strong antioxidant properties and its ability to help reduce skin damage caused by the sun.

Musk Splash

Aubrey Organics® herbal musk, a natural fragrance, contains no animal byproducts. (Also see Fragrances.)

Neem Oil

Neem trees grow in all parts of India, and are considered sacred by the Hindus, who use various parts of the tree in religious rituals and ceremonies. The bark, leaves and fruits of the neem have been used in ayurvedic (Hindu) medicine for thousands of years, and are mentioned in the ancient Sanskrit writings of Shushruta. The very name of the tree, nimba, is synonymous with Arishta, meaning "relief of sickness." The bark is a bitter tonic and astringent, used to lower fevers, as well as in the treatment of many skin diseases.

Washes, ointments and liniments for skin problems and ulcers are made from the leaves of the tree. In India various medical practitioners have successfully treated persistent skin ailments, some as serious as leprosy, with neem-based preparations. Applied as an oil or cream to fingernails, it appears to strengthen them and make them less likely to split or break.

Neem oil makes an excellent treatment for problem hair and scalp, particularly when combined with rosemary and sage oils. Used as a rinse or shampoo, it has proven effective in controlling stubborn cases of dandruff and other scalp disorders.

Nettle
(See Horsetail, Coltsfoot and Nettle)

Orange Blossom Oil

Essential oil used primarily as a flavoring agent and natural fragrance. (See Fragrances.)

Oregano Oil (Wild Marjoram)

Because this herb is considered a spice, especially in Italian cooking, it is often overlooked as a medicinal herb. Oregano has two major phenols *(thymol* and *carvacrol),* which have strong fungicidal and antiirritant properties. In European folk medicine it has been used in the treatment of spider bites, and in China it is added to preparations for the relief of itchy skin. I have used it successfully in a formula for topical yeast infections (Formula #27, "Yeast-Away" Anti-Yeast and Itch Prevention Cream). A drop of oregano oil in a glass of juice daily is also very helpful in the treatment of *Candida albicans.*

PABA

PABA, or para-aminobenzoic acid, is a water-soluble B vitamin found in bran, wheat germ, brewer's yeast, blackstrap molasses, eggs and organ meats. A well-known natural sunscreen, it offers a high degree of protection from harmful UV rays, especially when combined with other sun care herbals such as jojoba oil, shea butter, green tea and aloe vera.

Studies suggest that preparations containing PABA combined with selenium, the amino acid cysteine and the B vitamins inositol, biotin, pantothenic acid, folic acid and niacin can retard hair loss and help prevent graying. Used in shampoos, conditioners and hair gels, PABA will prevent damage of the disulfide bond in the hair, a leading cause of hair loss and breakage.

Though some allergic reactions to synthetic forms of PABA have been reported, we find that using food-grade, natural PABA in a vegetable glycerine base is well tolerated by most people with skin and scalp sensitivities.

Panthenol

Panthenol, also known as pantothenic acid or vitamin B-5, is a water soluble, B-complex vitamin found in a great number of sources, including bran, brewer's yeast, broccoli, brown rice, carrots, cheese, eggs, fish, legumes, wheat germ, whole grains and organ meats, particularly liver.

Combined with PABA, folic acid and inositol, it is one of the B vitamins reputed to help prevent gray hair. Panthenol also works beautifully as a hair thickener, and makes an excellent ingredient in natural hairsprays and styling gels, as well as shampoos that "add body" to thin, limp hair. Very little—if any—gums or resins are needed in a hairstyling product that contains panthenol. It is also an excellent skin hydrator, often found in moisturizers, lotions and complexion sprays. (See also Vitamins: B-Complex in this section, and Pantothenic Acid in Part III.)

Papain

An enzyme found in green papayas, papain is frequently recommended as an aid for digestion, and is a natural meat tenderizer. It is used in cosmetics as a skin softener.

Pectin

Found naturally in apples, bananas, beets, carrots, peas and other fruits and vegetables, pectin slows the absorption of food after a meal, which makes it an ideal digestive aid for people with diabetes. A strong antitoxic, it is sometimes used to reduce the side effects of radiation therapy. A natural thickener, it is used in cosmetics as an emulsifier.

Peppermint Oil

There are three major mints—peppermint, cornmint and spearmint— aromatic herbs used for both their taste and fragrance. Peppermint, the most popular one, has an important place in cosmetics. An antiseptic and astringent, peppermint oil is also a powerful antiinflammatory, used in massage creams and lotions, and in shampoos and hair rinses for its soothing effect on problem scalp. Its cooling and warming properties make it an excellent ingredient in therapeutic bath oils to relieve muscle aches and tension.

Perrier® Sparkling Mineral Water

Carbonated mineral water drawn from a naturally occurring source in Vergeze, the south of France. It contains traces of calcium, magnesium and bicarbonate. We use it as a refreshing base for our skin-revitalizing facial spray.

Pine Essential Oil

Extracted from the needles of Dwarf, Scotch, Siberian and other varieties of pine, this aromatic essential oil has antimicrobial and skin-purifying properties. It is frequently used as a fragrance. (See also Fragrances.)

ProGreens®

One of the richest, nutritionally whole foods formulas, ProGreens® (a trademark of NutriCology, Inc.) is a nutrient-dense blend of organic alfalfa, barley, oat and wheat grass juice in powdered form, combined with wheat sprouts, blue green and sea algae, lecithin, bioflavonoid extracts, royal jelly, bee pollen, vitamin E and other natural herbs and plant extracts.

We use ProGreens® in some of our cosmetic formulas for its nourishing and revitalizing properties when applied topically. Taken internally, it is a superb nutritional supplement. (Add one level scoop [8.8 g.] to 8 oz. of juice or water, and drink every morning on an empty stomach for best results.)

Psyllium Husks Powder

An active fiber that promotes digestion, psyllium husks powder is a good intestinal cleanser when taken internally. (Recommended adult dosage is 1 tsp. mixed in juice or water one to three times daily.) In cosmetic formulas, it is used to make hair and skin care gels.

Quick Oats

Quick Oats is organic and can be purchased at a health food store. It is used in facial masks. (See Formula #8, Meal & Herbs & Flowers Facial Scrub for All Skin Types.)

Quince Seed

The dried seeds of the quince, the fruit of a small tree belonging to the rose family. They are used in cosmetics as a thickener and emulsifier. An excellent natural hairspray can be made from quince seeds combined with grain alcohol or water.

Rice Cream

Rice cream, rice oil and rice powder are all great "smoothers" that improve the texture of a cosmetic formula naturally, without synthetic chemicals. As usual, buying organic is best.

Rosa Mosqueta® Rose Hip Seed Oil

The rare mountain rose that grows in the South American Andes is designated *Rosa rubiginosa*, but the natives call it Rosa Mosqueta, and have used the oil extracted from its rose hips for hundreds of years for its healing and skin-regenerating properties. This oil is rich in antioxidants, including vitamin C, carotenoids, flavonoids and polyphenols (one of the active ingredients in green tea), but perhaps its greatest benefit for the skin and scalp lies in its high concentration of essential fatty acids, particularly linoleic and linolenic acids, necessary for skin cell regeneration. (Its high content of essential fatty acids makes Rosa Mosqueta® oil comparable to evening primrose oil.)

Used straight or in skin care preparations, this ultra-moisturizing oil soothes flaking or irritated skin on contact, promotes healing and has been proven to help fade or prevent scarring and skin discolorations with continued use. In 1978, studies conducted by Dr. Fabiola Carvajal, M.D., at the University of Concepción in Santiago, Chile, showed Rosa Mosqueta® oil, when applied to severely burned patients, greatly reduced scarring and helped their skin heal at an amazing rate.

As rich an emollient as you'll ever find, Rosa Mosqueta® oil also works fast to improve skin texture, reverse sun damage and reduce the appearance of fine lines and wrinkles. Dermatological tests have proven that after a three-month daily application of the oil, patients showed diminished wrinkles, and lines around the mouth and eyes became much less noticeable. While it is not recommended for people actively suffering from acne, Rosa Mosqueta® oil was also successful in reducing the appearance of some acne scars. Further tests by radiologist and oncologist Dr. Hans Harbst also concluded that the oil can be used successfully in the treatment of scarring, inflammation and skin irritation caused by radiation therapy.

The examples of skin improvements using Rosa Mosqueta® oil and cream seem almost miraculous, but when combined with other anti-aging herbals, the results can be even more astonishing. Our cream made with Rosa Mosqueta®, aloe vera, green tea and white camellia and jojoba oils compounded into a tofu cream base is one of the finest antiwrinkle moisturizers you'll ever find at any price. But don't take our word for it. Turn to Formula #11 and see for yourself!

Rosemary

The famous quote from Shakespeare's Hamlet, "There's rosemary, that's for remembrance" is based on the idea that rosemary is good for the brain and the memory, and current research is examining its value in the treatment and prevention of Alzheimer's disease. This unique herbal also has a religious history. Rosemary was used by the ancients in place of more costly incense in religious ceremonies, and was considered a safeguard against witches and evil in Spain and Italy.

Both as an essential oil and a water extract, rosemary is an excellent hair and skin tonic and purifier. Used in hair products, it promotes circulation to scalps poorly supplied with blood, and is said to renew activity in dormant hair-bulbs to encourage growth and help prevent premature baldness. Combined with sage, rosemary makes an excellent hair rinse, and its mild, pleasant fragrance makes it an ideal ingredient in hair and skin care products.

Rosewater

Water-based dilution of the essence of roses, first prepared by Arab physician Avicenna in the 10th century. French rosewater and Bulgarian rosewater are superior to any developed elsewhere.

Rose Oil

The rose was probably cultivated in Persia and brought to Mesopotamia and across Asia Minor, and eventually into Greece and Italy. Rosa means "red" in Greek (from the word "rodon"), which suggests the Greek myth that the crimson-colored rose sprang from the blood of Adonis.

Scientific study of the rose has been mostly limited to improving the odor and appearance of the flower, rather than for the medicinal or cosmetic properties of its oil. Light yellow in color, rose oil has a strong scent of fresh roses and is generally included as a fragrance component in soaps, creams, lotions and perfumes. A water-based dilution of rose oil and vegetable glycerine makes a great skin softener.

Rose oils in general can't be synthetically produced. Even a supposedly artificial rose oil must contain some amount of natural rose oil in the formula. The natural oil should be used sparingly for a pleasant fragrance; too much of it is overpowering. It is excellent for "covering up" unpleasant odors in cosmetic products.

Royal Jelly

Royal jelly is a substance secreted in the digestive tube of the worker bees and eaten by the male and worker bees for a few days, and by the queen bee for her entire life (thus its name). A powerful nutrient with a full range of amino acids, minerals and enzymes, as well as vitamins A, B, C and E, and pantothenic acid, it has long been a part of Chinese medicine, usually mixed with tonic herbs, such as ginseng. Royal jelly has a soothing and moisturizing action on the skin.

Sage

Sage is much more than a tasty spice for your Thanksgiving turkey—it is an excellent hair and skin care ingredient. Sage, like rosemary, has a strong antioxidant action on the body. It is said to have antibacterial, antifungal and antiviral properties, and is mild enough to be nonirritating to even the most sensitive skin. A superb natural astringent, purifier and tonic, it is ideal for hair and scalp preparations. We combine it with rosemary to create some wonderful hair care products.

Sandalwood Oil

The oil from the sandalwood tree, an evergreen native to tropical Asia, is obtained by coarsely powdering, then steam- or water-distilling the heart wood, which yields 3% to 5% oil. This extremely expensive oil lends its distinctive fragrance to all kinds of cosmetics, and is frequently used in products for men.

Seasoap

Unique soap-in-a-jar formula from Aubrey Organics® used as a base in some of the soap and shampoo recipes. Its special blend of nutrient-rich seaweed extracts compounded into a mild castile and vegetable glycerine soap is very soothing to the skin, and rinses clean, without an oily residue. It also contains allantoin, shea butter and almond oil, three superb emollients to keep skin from drying out, and refreshing peppermint oil to freshen and purify. (See Formula #15, Lavender Liquid Body Soap.)

Selenium

A micro-mineral discovered in the earth's crust nearly 200 years ago, selenium is very effective in the treatment of dandruff and problem scalp. In addition to its scalp-clearing properties, selenium has been documented in several monographs and books as an aid to maintaining youthful skin and tissue elasticity (we like to call this the anti-aging factor), as well as for its antioxidant action, which helps neutralize certain cancer-causing free radicals in the body.

Though selenium is readily available in food, it is easily destroyed by food processing techniques. Adding synthetic chemicals will change its structure and eliminate its nutritional value. Selenium is even more valuable a nutrient when combined with vitamin E—these two antioxidants working together are much more powerful than the sum of their parts.

Besides helping control dandruff and itching, selenium has been found to reduce the age-related loss of hair pigment (or graying) caused by damage to the melanocytes (pigment cells) in the hair follicles. It has not been established whether its topical application in conditioners and shampoos will help maintain one's natural hair color, but selenium supplements taken internally have been shown to slow down the graying process. Hair care products that contain selenium can be slightly drying to the hair and scalp, so it is advisable to use it in small amounts and add herbal emollients to counteract this effect. In addition, be sure to follow with a good hair conditioner.

Shea Butter (Karite Butter)

Although it has not been extensively used in cosmetics, we have been adding shea butter (also known as karite butter or African butter) to our natural products for many years. I first learned about it when a man working for Sederma, a company in Meudon, France, sent me a jar to try in various formulations. I took just a bit on the tips of my fingers and applied it to the back of my hand. It was amazing how soft it made the skin, without leaving a greasy feel.

It is called African butter because it comes from a tree that grows in Central Africa. Natives gather the tiny, almond-like berries and extract the greenish-yellow buttery substance, which they use in cooking and in cosmetic preparations as a moisturizer and skin softener. (In Japan it is a popular substitute for regular dairy butter.)

Any plant oil or fat is mostly made up of esters of glycerol and saturated fatty acids. Another, smaller component is a group of substances called unsaponifiables. Unsaponifiable means that the substance can't be decomposed into an acid, alcohol or salt, which makes it very beneficial to the skin. Soybean and avocado oils are often used in cosmetics for their moisturizing and skin softening properties because they both have relatively high amounts of unsaponifiables. The exciting news about shea butter is that it has a higher amount of unsaponifiables than any other oil we use. Unsaponifiables are also responsible for shea butter's excellent spreadability and almost instant absorption into the skin.

Shea butter also contains a high amount of stigmasterol, a sterol known as the "anti-stiffness factor," which has long been used in Africa with astonishing results as a massage balm for tired, sore muscles and rheumatism, as well as in the treatment of household burns and minor wounds. The butter has a nourishing effect and seems to induce a state of self-protection in the cells. Clinical studies suggest that shea butter increases local capillary circulation, which in turns increases the amount of oxygen in tissues and stimulates the elimination of toxins from the body.

Another asset of this rich butter lies in its protective action when used in sunscreen formulations. Tests show that shea butter offers a high level of protection from the sun's harmful UV rays and prevents burning. Its high linoleic acid content makes it ideal for soothing dry or irritated skin, sunburn and chapping.

I have used shea butter in sun protection products, in soaps, moisturizers, antiwrinkle and celltherapy creams, in massage lotions and lip balms and, because it is a nontoxic and gentle ingredient, in baby and extra-sensitive skin products. You should be able to obtain a good quality shea or karite butter from your health food store and use it as an emollient in your own natural formulas.

Soybean Oil

An excellent emollient, soybean oil is very high in linoleic, oleic, linolenic and palmitic acids, essential fatty acids necessary for skin cell regeneration. (See Essential Fatty Acids.)

Spearmint Oil

One of the more popular mints, spearmint is most commonly used as a flavoring agent, but it is a wonderful skin tonic and purifier, with properties similar to peppermint oil. We use it in our toners, astringents and cleansers for its cooling and disinfecting effect on the skin.

St. John's Wort

An excellent emollient and skin softener, this healing herb is very beneficial to rough, damaged or irritated skin and problem scalp. It is particularly effective in suncare and after sun creams and lotions, and in cosmetic preparations for extremely sensitive, allergy-prone skin. Both the flowers and the oil extract have been used externally in the treatment of a wide variety of ailments. Its strong inflammation-inhibiting and nerve-soothing properties make it an ideal ingredient in ointments for arthritis and other joint disorders, as well as in the treatment of bruises, sprained muscles and minor cuts and burns.

Tea Tree Oil

Tea tree essential oil is distilled from the leaves of the *Malaleuca alterniforia*, a tree that grows only in the northeastern corner of Australia, where it has been successfully used for over 50 years in the treatment of many common skin disorders. The medicinal properties of this oil are similar to those of eucalyptus oil—both are known antiseptics and antimicrobials, and when added to hot water and inhaled, both soothe sore throats and help relieve sinus congestion. Many times more powerful than carbolic acid, tea tree oil can also be used to treat insect bites and stings, fungal conditions and minor skin infections.

Due to its strong odor, tea tree oil is not often added to cosmetics, but when used in tiny amounts and mixed with other essential oils to mask the smell, it makes an excellent ingredient for dandruff shampoos and therapeutic facial masks and creams.

Tea tree oil is an excellent ingredient in shampoos for oily or dry hair, depending on the preparation. For persons with dry hair, a 2% solution of tea tree oil added to a moisturizing shampoo will help unblock sebaceous glands and encourage the free flow of the body's own oils, while clearing away dead skin cells in the scalp. For people with oily hair, a gentle tea tree oil shampoo will cleanse the scalp of bacterial and fungal irritations and help dislodge dead skin cells. A few drops of tea tree oil rubbed into the scalp will also help regulate overly dry or oily scalp, relieve itching and help control dandruff.

Tea tree oil has also proven effective in treatments against head lice, a common affliction among school children which can be hard to eradicate. In Part V we feature recipes for two hair care products that contain tea tree oil, Blue Green Algae Hair Rescue Mask and Blue Green Algae Hair Rescue Shampoo (Formulas #21 and #20), which have been successful in treating head lice. Soaking combs, brushes and other contaminated materials in a solution of three drops of tea tree oil in one pint of alcohol is also highly recommended when treating head lice, as this will guard against reinfection.

Natural tea tree oil has many topical uses and has proven effective in relieving or clearing up the following ailments:

For athlete's foot and other fungal foot conditions, and to help control unpleasant foot odors: Try our Feet Rescue Cream for Troubled Feet (Formula #28 in Part V).

For nail fungi and/or infections: Soak fingernails or toenails in pure tea tree oil, massaging the solution into the nail bed twice daily until infection clears.

For diaper rash: Add six drops of tea tree oil to our Natural Baby's Evening Primrose Lotion (Formula #30) and use on baby twice a day as needed.

For babies' cradle cap: Add six drops of tea tree oil to our Natural Baby's Evening Primrose Shampoo (Formula #29) and use daily. Note: Be sure not to get the shampoo in baby's eyes, as tea tree oil will burn.

Tofu

Over 4,000 years ago the Chinese discovered the value of the soybean as a source of protein. By the 1920s, farmers in the U.S. had begun to grow soybean crops in commercial quantities, and today more soybeans are cultivated in the U.S. than anywhere else. The soybean converts nutrients from the soil into quality, edible protein with incredible efficiency, and is the largest nutritive source of both protein and oil in the world. Soy protein is acknowledged to be the highest quality form of vegetable protein and is also one of the most abundant.

For the past 30 years, the soyfood market in America has hosted more than 2,000 new products since 1985, all in response to the increasing demand for a healthier alternative to meat and dairy products, a desire to reduce intake of animal fats, and the growing popularity of vegetarianism. Soyfoods come in many shapes and forms, with something for everyone: tofu, tempeh, soymilk, sprouts, flour and nuts.

Of all the soyfood eaten, tofu is the most common. A quarter pound of tofu contains 9 grams of protein (twice that of fish and white meats), 145 mg. calcium and 4.1 mg. iron. It also contains phosphorus, potassium, B-complex vitamins (particularly choline) and vitamin E. It is, as you can see, an excellent nutrient for the hair, scalp and skin.

I have used soy protein in my cosmetic products for over two decades, and have found that my tofu cream base is one of the best absorption bases you can find, far superior to cream bases in most commercial hair and skin care products. (To make a simple version of this base, see Formula #1, Natural Absorption Base.)

Vegetable Glycerine
A rich humectant, emollient and lubricant naturally extracted from vegetable oils, glycerine has been used in cosmetic formulations for thousands of years. Synthetic glycerine, derived from propylene glycol, is highly irritating to the skin and scalp and should be avoided.

Vegetable Protein
Known as "the building block of life," protein is our most important food, a leading source of vitamins and amino acids. Generally found in meat, eggs and dairy products, protein can also be obtained from soya, wheat, almond, certain microalgae (including blue green algae and spirulina) and other sources. Applied topically, vegetable protein is an excellent hydrator, readily absorbed by the skin. In hair care formulas, it combines with essential fatty acids and amino acids to coat porous or damaged hair and help repair split ends.

Vitamins
Vitamins are biologically active substances essential for all physiological functions in the body. They are considered biocatalysts—that is, they act as mediators of biochemical processes in the body without actually taking part in the processes themselves.

Vitamins have to be supplied from outside, since the body is not able to synthesize them. A vitamin deficiency, as we discussed earlier, leads not only to internal disorders, but can also cause characteristic damage to the hair, skin and nails. These deficiencies are usually treated by oral supplementation. However, clinical studies have shown that topical application of vitamins results in a higher concentration of vitamins in the skin than can be obtained by taking them orally. Thus, treating the skin externally with vitamins by adding them to your cosmetic products just makes good sense. (For a more in-depth discussion of vitamins and vitamin deficiencies, see Part III, Diet, Nutrition and Your Hair and Skin.)

We include many vitamins in our formulas, either as ingredients or as components of an herb or plant extract. Here's a brief rundown of some important vitamins and what they can do for your hair and skin:

– Vitamin A –
This fat-soluble vitamin may have more cosmetic uses than any other vitamin you can put on your skin. Used topically, vitamin A promotes the formation of new skin cells and stimulates oil secretion in the sebaceous glands without increasing it above normal. It has also been shown to help clear up some forms of acne, both in topical applications and taken orally (particularly when combined with zinc), and to relieve symptoms of psoriasis and other skin disorders. Beneficial to dry or damaged skin, it is often found in sun protection creams for its healing and hydrating properties. A version of vitamin A—retinoic acid (also called vitamin A acid)—is classified as a drug, and has proven effective as an acne treatment, although it causes allergic

reactions in some people. (See also Carrot Oil.)

– Vitamin B-Complex –

The vitamins of the B series regulate many metabolic processes, and thus have a great significance for the body. B vitamins, mainly found in yeast and grains, have a particularly beneficial effect on the skin, hair and nails.

The absence of these vitamins—the most important being B-1, B-2, B-6 and B-12—triggers some serious functional disturbances in the body, and often is reflected in poor conditions of the skin, hair and nails. Certain skin disorders, such as seborrheic dermatitis, excessive oil secretion and flaking and scaling of the skin and scalp can be directly related to B-vitamin deficiencies.

It has been clinically shown that certain B vitamins are also absorbed by the skin and take effect there, so that topical application of them is important. It's interesting to note that the group of vitamin B factors are shown to be much more effective as a unit—that is, as a "complex"—than they would be when taken or applied individually. It is better to use a B-complex vitamin prepared from natural, raw materials since, in addition to the B vitamins themselves, such a complex contains other companion substances found in nature that work synergistically to help the body absorb and metabolize these nutrients more effectively. Nutritional yeast and brewer's yeast are excellent sources of total-complex B vitamins.

– Vitamin C –

Vitamin C is ascorbic acid plus a complex of other factors (rutin, hesperidin and other bioflavonoids) present in fresh foods, especially citrus fruits. This antioxidant vitamin makes an excellent natural preservative in cosmetics, both in the water phase and oil phase (particularly in its fat-soluble form, ascorbyl palmitate). Vitamin C plays an essential role in building collagen, the connective tissue that holds us together. The bioflavonoids help promote the effectiveness of vitamin C and help build capillary strength. A new and more stable form of vitamin C, called Ester-C®, is now available in health food stores. (U.S. Patent by Inter-Cal, Inc.)

– Vitamin E –

Vitamin E is one of the best known antioxidants in use, protecting the body from free radical damage caused by sun exposure and environmental pollutants. Vitamin E may be natural or synthetic; if natural, it comes from vegetable sources. (We recommend you use only natural vitamin E in your formulas.)

Vitamin E lends itself to the preventive care of every type of skin. Studies show topically applied preparations containing this fat-soluble vitamin improve blood circulation to the skin and scalp, promote skin cell regeneration and strengthen the connective tissue in the skin. Age-related symptoms of connective tissue degeneration in the skin also respond well to vitamin E therapy.

Vitamin E works well as a preservative in the oil phase of cosmetics, particularly when combined with vitamins C and A. Used in cosmetic preparations, it helps keep the products stable and prevents deterioration from oxidation and the growth of bacteria, protecting the oils in lotions, shampoos and creams from becoming rancid.

– Vitamin F –
(See Essential Fatty Acids)

Wheat Germ Oil, Wheat Germ Extract

Wheat germ is the embryo of the wheat berry. A superb source of nutrients, both the powdered extract and the oil are extremely high in vitamins, essential fatty acids, minerals and trace minerals. At the top of the list of benefits is its high content of vitamin E, a powerful antioxidant that inhibits the oxidation processes in the body and protects it against harmful free radicals. (See Vitamin E entry on previous page.) Other substances found in both wheat germ oil and extract include provitamin A, B vitamins, lecithin and sterols.

One problem lies in the fact that wheat germ becomes rancid easily, so make sure the product is vacuum packed or refrigerated, and look for a packing date or expiration date on the container. Because heat and/or chemicals break down the structure of its nutrients, only cold pressed wheat germ oil should be used.

We will be formulating only with the powdered extract. To use powdered wheat germ in your cosmetic formulas, combine one heaping teaspoon of powder with 1/4 cup 150 proof natural grain alcohol and 1/4 cup of vegetable glycerine.

White Camellia Oil

This rich oil has been hand-harvested in the villages of China and Japan for hundreds of years and used topically for its soothing and moisturizing properties. It's not only excellent for the skin, but works wonders on the hair as well. We include it in many of our hair and skin care products, including an ultra-moisturizing shampoo and a spray-on, non-greasy conditioner for dull-looking hair. High in essential fatty acids and vitamins A, B and E, this superb emollient and nutrient is featured in several of our recipes.

Willowherb, Canadian

An antiirritant and antiinflammatory, Canadian willowherb is an excellent treatment for itching, flaking or irritated skin. Applied topically, it soothes and smooths the skin, and has antiseptic and detoxifying properties. Clinical tests conducted among men and women 18 to 60 years old showed a willowherb-based cream was found more effective than a 1% hydrocortisone cream in reducing itching, redness and irritation of the skin. Within 30 minutes of the willowherb cream application, 25% of the patients showed improvement, while only 15% of the patients using the hydrocortisone cream showed some improvement.

This study points to the fact that willowherb may not only be the superior treatment, but it is a much safer one, since continuous use of hydrocortisone, a powerful steroid, can break down the skin's collagen over time, and long term absorption into the body may lead to hormonal imbalances and other problems. Canadian willowherb has no known side effects, and may do a better job of relieving the symptoms of eczema, psoriasis and other skin disorders than many medicated creams on the market.

Wintergreen Oil

A tonic and astringent, wintergreen oil's warming action on the skin makes it an ideal ingredient for massage lotions, sports rubs and therapeutic bath oils. One of its components, gaultherin, is made up of 90% methyl salicylate, a substance similar to aspirin, which gives wintergreen oil pain relieving and antiinflammatory properties. An aromatic essential oil, it is often used as a flavoring, and as a fragrance in cosmetics.

Witch Hazel

Witch hazel is probably the most recognized skin purifier in the plant world. Witch hazel leaf, witch hazel bark and witch hazel water (also known as hamamelis water or distilled witch hazel extract) have all been reported to have astringent and skin-freshening properties.

Witch hazel preparations are made from the dried leaves, bark and twigs of a shrub native to North America. Witch hazel water, a milder extract, is obtained from the recently cut and partially dried twigs, which are soaked for 24 hours in twice their weight in warm water, then are distilled. A small amount of alcohol (15% or less) is then added to the distillate and thoroughly mixed.

Both the pharmaceutical and cosmetic industries use witch hazel extract in dozens of preparations—from suppositories and ointments to baby wipes, mouthwashes and shaving lotions. The bottled witch hazel sold in drug stores is simply witch hazel water, the most common of the three preparations, and can be used in the cosmetics you create. It is an excellent ingredient for skin care, particularly when combined with soothing aloe vera. An important and sometimes overlooked topical ingredient, it's an excellent herbal to rediscover.

Yucca Root

An excellent skin and hair purifier, yucca root is used in soaps and shampoos for its gentle lathering and cleansing properties. It contains saponins, naturally occurring glycosides that foam in water to create a mild, natural detergent. Yucca root also has antiinflammatory properties, and is used medicinally in the treatment of arthritis and other inflammatory disorders.

For a full overview of how certain herbs can work for you, we've prepared a chart (see following pages) which puts at your fingertips a lot of valuable information on both their topical and internal use. This easy-to-use reference will be helpful whether you're making your own cosmetic products or reading cosmetic labels in your health food store.

Topical Applications of Herbs

	Astringent	Calmative	Cleansing	Circulation of (internal/external)	Cuts, bruises, skin, massage	Eczema, acne, skin disorders	Inflammation	Moisturizing, softening	Muscle tension	Pain relief	Rejuvenation	Soothing qualities	Stimulant	Veins, capillaries
AGRIMONY	●				●	●	●	●		●	●	●		
ALOE					●	●	●	●						
ALMONDS								●						
ALTHEA ROOT	●							●				●		
ANGELICA		●												
APRICOT								●						
ARAROBA (GOA)	●					●								
ARISTOLOCHIA					●		●				●	●		
ARNICA				●	●			●					●	
AVOCADO				●		●		●						
BALM OF GILEAD					●								●	
BALSAM OF PERU	●		●					●						
BALSAM TOLU	●		●					●						
BEARSFOOT													●	
BEDSTRAW	●		●		●	●							●	

	Astringent	Calmative	Cleansing	Circulation of (internal/external)	Cuts, bruises, skin, massage	Eczema, acne, skin disorders	Inflammation	Moisturizing, softening	Muscle tension	Pain relief	Rejuvenation	Soothing qualities	Stimulant	Veins, capillaries
BENZOIN	●					●								
BERGAMOT OIL						●								
BETULLA	●													
BISTORT	●			●										
BLADDERWRACK			●	●				●				●		
BONESET				●		●							●	
BORAGE					●		●	●			●	●		
BUTCHERS BROOM	●													
CADE OIL					●	●								
CAJEPUT OIL	●												●	
CALAMUS, SWEET FLAG			●											
CALENDULA (Marigold)	●		●	●	●	●	●	●	●	●		●		●
CAMOMILE	●	●	●		●		●	●		●		●		
CAMPHOR	●						●					●	●	
CATHECHU (Black/Pale)	●													
CENTAURY	●	●										●		
CHAULMOOGRA		●			●	●	●							
CINNAMON	●													

Property	GOLDEN ROD	GINSENG	GINGER	GERANIUM	FRANKINCENSE	FENNEL	EYEBRIGHT	EVENING PRIMROSE	EUCALYPTUS	ELECAMPANE	ELDER FLOWERS	ECHINACEA	DANDELION	CUCUMBER	COWSLIP	COMFREY	COLTSFOOT	COCOA
Astringent		•		•			•	•	•	•	•			•		•		
Calmative	•	•					•								•			
Cleansing	•			•		•	•	•	•	•			•	•		•	•	
Circulation of (internal/external)			•						•							•		
Cuts, bruises, skin, massage												•				•	•	
Eczema, acne, skin disorders						•		•		•			•			•		
Inflammation																•		
Moisturizing, softening		•		•				•		•				•		•		•
Muscle tension										•								
Pain relief																•		
Rejuvenation						•							•			•		
Soothing qualities														•		•		
Stimulant		•	•		•						•		•					
Veins, capillaries																•		

	Astringent	Calmative	Cleansing	Circulation of (internal/external)	Cuts, bruises, skin, massage	Eczema, acne, skin disorders	Inflammation	Moisturizing, softening	Muscle tension	Pain relief	Rejuvenation	Soothing qualities	Stimulant	Veins, capillaries
GOLDENSEAL	•					•								
GRAPEFRUIT OIL			•			•								
GREATER CELANDINE			•			•								
HAWTHORN	•													
HEARTSEASE						•								
HENNA														
HOPS								•						
HORSE CHESTNUT	•			•										
HORSETAIL	•	•	•		•	•				•				
HYSSOP					•	•								
IMMORTELLE					•	•		•						
IVY		•		•				•				•		
JASMINE		•												
JUNIPER BERRIES	•		•			•								
KELP				•										
LADY'S MANTLE	•		•		•									
LAVENDER	•	•	•	•	•	•	•	•	•		•	•		
LICORICE ROOT							•							

Property	ROSEMARY	RHATONY	ROSA MOSQUETA	RAMSONS	QUILLAIA	PLANTAIN, RIBWORT	PIPSISSEWA	PARIS HERB	PAPAIN	ORANGE OIL (BLOSSOM)	OLIVE OIL	OATS	NETTLE	MYRRH	MUSK SEED	MISTLETOE	MALLOW, BLUE	LINDEN TREE
Astringent		●					●			●	●		●	●				
Calmative												●			●	●		●
Cleansing	●			●	●	●	●		●		●	●		●		●	●	●
Circulation of (internal/external)	●									●					●			
Cuts, bruises, skin, massage			●			●			●							●		
Eczema, acne, skin disorders	●				●	●	●	●	●		●				●	●		
Inflammation			●		●	●			●	●								
Moisturizing, softening		●	●						●	●	●		●				●	●
Muscle tension	●																	
Pain relief			●													●	●	
Rejuvenation	●	●	●						●	●								●
Soothing qualities			●					●										●
Stimulant												●	●					
Veins, capillaries	●		●							●								

Herb	Astringent	Calmative	Cleansing	Circulation of (internal/external)	Cuts, bruises, skin, massage	Eczema, acne, skin disorders	Inflammation	Moisturizing, softening	Muscle tension	Pain relief	Rejuvenation	Soothing qualities	Stimulant	Veins, capillaries
RUTIN														•
SAGE			•				•							
SHEPHERD'S PURSE		•	•		•	•		•	•	•				
SPEEDWELL		•	•		•					•			•	
STINGING NETTLE			•	•	•	•				•			•	
ST. JOHN'S WORT	•			•		•	•	•				•		•
STORAX	•					•								
STRAWBERRY	•					•								
SUNFLOWER OIL			•	•										
THYME		•	•		•									
WALNUT			•		•	•								
WILLOW (Small Flowered)			•											
WINTERGREEN OIL	•		•	•					•			•	•	
WITCH HAZEL	•		•	•	•	•	•	•						•
WOOD SORREL			•			•								
YARROW			•	•			•	•				•		
YELLOW DEAD NETTLE			•			•						•		•

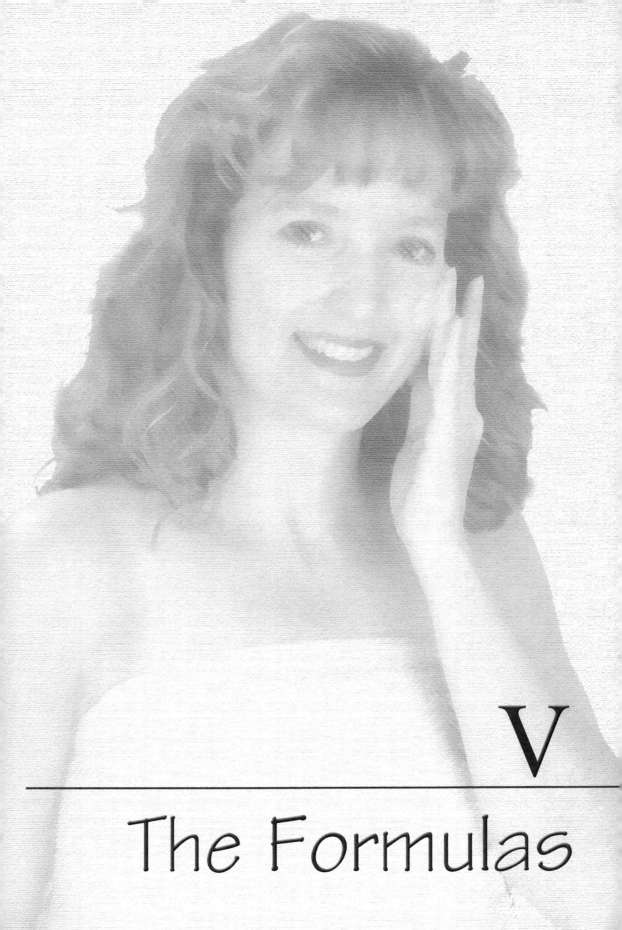

V

The Formulas

C ongratulations! You are about to become a gourmet cosmetic chef, right in
your own kitchen, and make some of the finest and most unique natural
cosmetics you'll ever find. The measuring chart below will help you with
any conversions you'll need to do. The formulas in this book are all written in kitchen
terms because that's how I first made them, in my own kitchen. Wade right in and
start creating your own creams, lotions, soaps, shampoos and more. But just remember, if you start selling these superb natural products, you'll have to give us a piece of
the action!

Equivalent Measures and Weights

LIQUID MEASURES

1 gal	=	4 qt	=	8 pt	=	16 cups	=	128 fl oz	=	3.79 L
1/2 gal	=	2 qt	=	4 pt	=	8 cups	=	64 fl oz	=	1.89 L
1/4 gal	=	1 qt	=	2 pt	=	4 cups	=	32 fl oz	=	.95 L
1/2 qt	=	1 pt	=	2 cups	=	16 fl oz	=	.47 L		
1/4 qt	=	1/2 pt	=	1 cup	=	8 fl oz	=	.24 L		

DRY MEASURES

1 cup	=	8 fl oz	=	16 tbsp	=	48 tsp	=	237 ml
3/4 cup	=	6 fl oz	=	12 tbsp	=	36 tsp	=	177 ml
2/3 cup	=	5 1/3 fl oz	=	10 2/3 tbsp	=	32 tsp	=	158 ml
1/2 cup	=	4 fl oz	=	8 tbsp	=	24 tsp	=	118 ml
1/3 cup	=	2 2/3 fl oz	=	5 1/3 tbsp	=	16 tsp	=	79 ml
1/4 cup	=	2 fl oz	=	4 tbsp	=	12 tsp	=	59 ml
1/8 cup	=	1 fl oz	=	2 tbsp	=	6 tsp	=	30 ml
1 tbsp	=	3 tsp	=	15 ml					

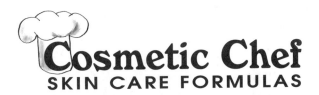

Cosmetic Chef
SKIN CARE FORMULAS

FORMULA #1
Natural Absorption Base

Aubrey's Tofu Essential Fatty Acid Cream Base

This essential fatty acid base will be the starting point of many of the
formulas you will be making. I first created this natural cold cream base
in the late 60s and have been using some version of it ever since in many
hair and skin care products. Absorption bases are an important part of a cosmetic
formula. They work as a "carrying agent"—that is, they help carry herbs, vitamins and other nutrients deep into the hair shaft, scalp and skin. Unlike most
absorption bases, which are a blend of lanolin, beeswax, mineral oil and various
other synthetic oils, my cream base contains only protein-rich tofu, natural plant
extracts and herbal oils high in essential fatty acids, necessary for the health of
your hair and skin.

Its greatest selling point is that, unlike mineral oil-based cold creams that can
stay on top of your skin, cause clogged pores and leave a greasy residue, this
cream base is absorbed almost instantly and can be used in all kinds of products
for all skin types. This formula is 100% vegan, which is another reason many
people will like it.

Here is a simple version of "The Base." Remember to use organic ingredients
whenever possible for best results.

INGREDIENTS:
Tofu (soft, silken, preferred brands: Mori-Nu, VitaSoy, Eden Foods) — 1 cup
Aloe Vera Gel (preferred brand: Aubrey Organics®, or fresh gel from aloe plant
    — just remove fillet from leaf and liquefy in blender) — 1/4 cup (4 Tbsp.)
Flaxseed Oil (preferred brands: Barleans, Arrowhead Mills) — 1 tsp.
Evening Primrose Oil (preferred brand: Aubrey Organics®) — 1/4 tsp.
Shea Butter (preferred brands: Frontier, Karite-One) — 1/4 cup (4 Tbsp.)
Natural Grain Alcohol (150 proof) — 1 Tbsp. *without*
Grapefruit Seed Extract (preferred brand: NutriBiotic) — 1/4 tsp.

HOW TO DO IT:
Drain tofu and place into a blender. Add the aloe vera gel, flaxseed oil, evening

primrose oil, grain alcohol, grapefruit seed extract and shea butter, then blend until uniform, being careful not to over-blend. Mixture should be smooth and thick. Put the base into an opaque container with a tight lid and keep it in the refrigerator until you're ready to use it.

HOW TO USE IT:

This cream base will be used as a carrying agent in many of the products you make. Keep some on hand in your refrigerator and use as needed in any of these formulas.

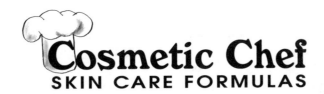

Cosmetic Chef
SKIN CARE FORMULAS

FORMULA #2
Aubrey's Herbal Base

This herbal base will be used in many of the skin care formulas you will be making, including astringents, moisturizers and exfoliating herbal masks. While obtaining all the individual herbs will seem like a big investment at first, you will find that once you've purchased them, you will be using them over and over in your recipes. All these herbals should be available in the bulk herbs section of your health food store.

INGREDIENTS:
Benzoin Gum — 2 Tbsp.
Calendula Blossoms (Marigolds) — 2 Tbsp.
Camomile Flowers — 3 Tbsp.
Coltsfoot Leaves — 1 Tbsp.
Comfrey Root— 1 Tbsp.
Echinacea — 1 Tbsp
Eucalyptus Leaves — 1 Tbsp.
Elder Berries — 2 Tbsp
Fennel — 1 Tbsp.
Horsetail — 1 Tbsp.
Lavender Flowers — 2 Tbsp.
Marshmallow Root — 2 Tbsp.
Nettle Leaves — 2 Tbsp.
Rosemary — 1 Tbsp.
Sage — 1 Tbsp.
St. John's Wort — 1 Tbsp.
Natural Grain Alcohol or triple distilled Vodka — 16 oz. (1 pint)
Distilled Water — 16 oz. (1 pint)

HOW TO DO IT:
Pour the grain alcohol or vodka into a clean container. Add the herbs and allow them to remain in the liquid for four hours or more. Next, pour herbs and

alcohol blend into a pint of boiling water and steep for 30 minutes. Finally, strain the mixture by pouring it through a clean towel, squeezing towel to get all the liquid.

HOW TO USE IT:

Store your herbal base in a clean container in the refrigerator until needed for the different formulas. As some of the recipes require a mixture of the dry herbals only, you may wish to combine the herbs beforehand, and not add the water or alcohol. Just store the herbal mixture in a plastic bag and keep it in a cool, dry place until you're ready to make your formulas.

Skin Care Products
Cleansers, Toners & Masks

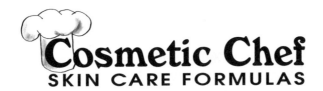

Cosmetic Chef
SKIN CARE FORMULAS

FORMULA #3
Natural Facial Cleansing Cream
For Normal, Oily or Problem Skin

This facial cleanser is similar to one we've been making for over 20 years, and it's the best formula around for oily, combination or acne-prone complexions. It goes to work instantly on your skin with the gentle medicinal action of herbal oils in a mild tofu and aloe base. Used regularly, it helps regulate excess oil production and clear and disinfect the skin to keep it smooth and blemish-free.

Be sure to follow this recipe exactly. Only drops of the various essential oils are called for in the mixture, which offers the therapeutic and skin-conditioning effects of the oils without making your skin too greasy. Though it is especially formulated for oily or acne-prone complexions, this cleanser is so gentle, we also recommend it for normal or combination skin.

INGREDIENTS:

Tofu (soft, preferred brands: Mori-Nu, VitaSoy, Eden Foods) — 1 cup
Aloe Vera Gel (preferred brand: Aubrey Organics®, or fresh gel from aloe plant
— just remove fillet from leaf and liquefy in blender) — 1 Tbsp.
Yucca Root Extract (preferred brand: Gaia) — 2/3 cup
Eucalyptus Oil (preferred brands: Aura Cacia, Frontier) — 2 drops
Peppermint Oil (preferred brands: Aura Cacia, Frontier, Gaia) — 2 drops
Spearmint Oil (preferred brands: Aura Cacia, Frontier, Gaia) — 2 drops
Sage Oil (preferred brands: Aura Cacia, Frontier, Gaia) — 2 drops
Rosemary Oil (preferred brands: Aura Cacia, Frontier, Gaia) — 2 drops
Tea Tree Oil (preferred brands: Aura Cacia, Desert Essence) — 2 drops
Camphor Oil (preferred brands: Aura Cacia, Frontier, Gaia) — 2 drops
Wintergreen Oil (preferred brands: Aura Cacia, Frontier, Gaia) — 2 drops
Lemon Oil (preferred brands: Aura Cacia, Frontier, Gaia) — 1/4 tsp.
Grapefruit Seed Extract (preferred brand: NutriBiotic) — 1/4 tsp.

HOW TO DO IT:

Place drained tofu into a blender. Add the yucca root extract and the aloe vera gel. With a dropper, add the essential oils in the order and amounts indicated, and hand stir into mixture. (Blend lightly, making sure not to over-mix.) When completed, the cleansing lotion should be semi-thick and light brown in color.

HOW TO USE IT:

Twice daily splash face with warm water, then slowly work cleanser over skin with fingers or washcloth, massaging lightly. Rinse thoroughly with warm water, and follow with a natural toner and moisturizer. IMPORTANT: Keep refrigerated when not in use.

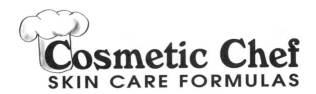

Cosmetic Chef
SKIN CARE FORMULAS

FORMULA #4
Natural Facial Cleansing Cream
For Normal to Dry Skin

T his formula differs from the previous cleanser (Natural Facial Cleansing Cream for Normal, Oily or Problem Skin) in that it contains several highly moisturizing essential oils to aid dry, lifeless or mature skin. It is based on a formula I created over 30 years ago, which is still one of the top-selling natural facial cleansers.

INGREDIENTS:
Tofu Fatty Acid Cream Base (See Formula #1) — 1 cup
Yucca Root Extract (preferred brands: Gaia, Pioneer) — 3/4 cup
White Camellia Oil (preferred brand: Aubrey Organics®) — 1/4 tsp.
Rosa Mosqueta® Rose Hip Seed Oil (available only from Aubrey Organics®) —
    1/4 tsp.
Milk Thistle Extract (preferred brands: Aura Cacia, Frontier, Gaia) — 1/4 tsp.
Shea Butter (preferred brands: Frontier, Karite-One) — 2 Tbsp.
Lemon Oil (preferred brands: Aura Cacia, Frontier, Gaia) — 1/4 tsp
Grapefruit Seed Extract (preferred brand: NutriBiotic) — 1/4 tsp.

HOW TO DO IT:
Place Tofu Fatty Acid Cream Base in a mixing bowl. Add the yucca root extract and stir. Next add the white camellia and Rosa Mosqueta® oils and continue stirring into mixture. (When you open the Rosa Mosqueta® and white camellia oils, you will need to pry off the applicator top on the bottle. To do this, simply grasp applicator firmly with fingers and pull it off.) Place shea butter in a small sauce pan on the stove and heat until it melts, then add it to mixture, stirring in slowly without over-mixing. Gently stir in the rest of the ingredients, adding the lemon oil and grapefruit seed extract last. The mixture should be semi-thick to thin, with a lotion-type consistency, and will be light brown in color. Place lotion into an applicator bottle and store in the refrigerator until you're ready to use it.

HOW TO USE IT:

Shake well before using. Dampen face with warm water, then apply a small amount of cleanser onto fingers or washcloth and work well over face, massaging lightly. Rinse with warm water, and follow with a natural toner and moisturizer. IMPORTANT: Keep refrigerated when not in use.

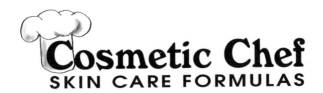

Cosmetic Chef
SKIN CARE FORMULAS

FORMULA #5
Rosa Mosqueta® & Lavender Herbal Toner
For Normal to Dry Skin

he purpose of any astringent or toner is twofold: it should clear the skin of soap residue and debris left after cleansing, and also work as a kind of "tonic" to stimulate skin circulation, smooth and freshen the complexion and prepare it for better absorption of a moisturizer. This important skin care step is often overlooked, yet people who use a facial toner regularly simply have healthier skin.

If your skin is dry, you probably have a hard time finding a good toner. Most commercial toners are strong astringents that contain alcohol and acetone, which are harsh and very drying, and often cause allergic reactions and irritation. This particular formula contains just enough essential oils to soothe and hydrate dry, mature or sensitive skin.

INGREDIENTS:
Witch Hazel (preferred brand: Dickenson's) — 1 cup
Shea Butter (preferred brands: Frontier, Karite-One) — 1 Tbsp.
Aubrey's Herbal Base (Formula #2) — 1/2 cup
Aloe Vera (preferred brand: Aubrey Organics®, or fresh gel from aloe plant — just remove fillet and liquefy in blender) — 2 Tbsp.
Rosa Mosqueta® Rose Hip Seed Oil (available only from: Aubrey Organics®) — 2 tsp.
Lavender Essential Oil (preferred brands: Tisserand, Gaia) — 8 drops
Vegetable Glycerine — 1/2 cup
Grapefruit Seed Extract (preferred brand: NutriBiotic) — 1/4 tsp.

HOW TO DO IT:
Pour 1/2 cup of Herbal Base (Formula #2) into a sauce pan. Add the vegetable glycerine, shea butter and Rosa Mosqueta® oil and heat gently until the

shea butter melts. Remove from heat, stir in the aloe vera, then add the grapefruit seed extract and the 4 drops of lavender oil. Pour the mixture slowly into the witch hazel while stirring. Place toner in a bottle and keep it refrigerated when not in use.

HOW TO USE IT:

Shake well before using. Clean skin with a good facial cleanser and pat dry. Then soak a cotton ball or pad with toner and wipe gently across face and neck in upward strokes, changing cotton as needed. Your skin will feel fresh, clear and soft—never tight or dry.

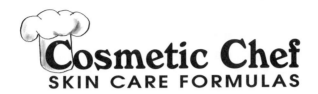

Cosmetic Chef
SKIN CARE FORMULAS

FORMULA #6
Aubrey's Herbal Facial Astringent
For Normal to Oily Skin

This astringent is very similar to another of my popular formulas that has been around for more than two decades. Through the years I've refined it and tested it on thousands of people with excellent results. It not only tones and disinfects the complexion, it also works to normalize the skin and break up dirt and oil deposits. (That's why astringents are sometimes known as "skin clarifiers.") You can keep your complexion clear and healthy-looking with this easy-to-make formula.

INGREDIENTS:

Aubrey's Herbal Base (Formula #2) — 7 oz.
Witch Hazel (preferred brand: Dickenson's) — 1/2 cup
Aloe Vera Gel (preferred brand: Aubrey Organics®, or fresh gel from aloe plant
     — just remove fillet from leaf and liquefy in blender) — 3 Tbsp.
Eucalyptus Oil (preferred brands: Aura Cacia, Frontier, Gaia) — 1 drop
Peppermint Oil (preferred brands: Aura Cacia, Frontier, Gaia) — 1 drop
Spearmint Oil (preferred brands: Aura Cacia, Frontier, Gaia) — 1 drop
Rosemary Oil (preferred brands: Aura Cacia, Frontier, Gaia) — 1 drop
Lemon Peel Oil (preferred brands: Aura Cacia, Frontier) — 1/4 tsp.
Grapefruit Seed Extract (preferred brand: NutriBiotic) — 1/4 tsp.

HOW TO DO IT:

Pour the Herbal Base (Formula #2) into a clean container and combine it with the witch hazel. Add the essential oils in order shown, then finish with the grapefruit seed extract. The astringent should be a light brown, the color of tea. IMPORTANT: Keep in the refrigerator when not in use.

HOW TO USE IT:

Shake well before using. After cleansing, soak cotton ball or pad with astringent and wipe gently across face and neck in upward strokes, changing cotton as needed. Follow with a good, natural moisturizer.

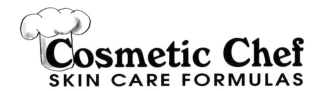

Cosmetic Chef
SKIN CARE FORMULAS

FORMULA #7
Green Clay & Blue Green Algae
Moisturizing Mask for All Skin Types

I **once mixed a batch of this mask** at Mrs. Gooch's Whole Foods Market in Sherman Oaks, California, during a shooting of *Good Day Los Angeles* for KTTV-TV (Fox). As I added the Green Kamut®, the blue green algae and the clay, the mixture became greener and greener. Jon Melichar, a very funny man who hosts the show on location, looked at the mixture and noted its strong resemblance to guacamole. Suddenly, he dipped a taco chip into the mask and ate it, an action he instantly regretted, judging from the sour look on his face!

Later we applied the green mask to Jon's face. He had donned a yellow zoot suit and hat for the occasion, which made him look just like Jim Carrey in *The Mask*. He smiled into the camera and said, "Smokin'!" Here's that very same deep-cleansing and skin-revitalizing mask. We recommend you put it on your face, not in your mouth.

INGREDIENTS:

Tofu Essential Fatty Acid Cream Base (see Formula #1) — 1 cup
Aloe Vera Fillet (preferred brand: Aubrey Organics® Out of the Leaf Aloe Vera
    Fillet, or use the fresh fillet from your own aloe plant) — 1 fillet
Green Kamut® (Green Kamut Corp.) — 7 Tbsp. (1/2 cup minus 1 Tbsp.)
Blue Green Algae Powder (preferred brand: Klamath) — 1 tsp.
French Green Clay (preferred brand: Rainbow Research) — 2 Tbsp.
Rosa Mosqueta® Rose Hip Seed Oil (available only from Aubrey Organics®) —
    1/4 tsp.
Evening Primrose Oil (preferred brand: Aubrey Organics®) — 1/4 tsp.
White Camellia Oil (preferred brand: Aubrey Organics®) — 1/4 tsp.
Grapefruit Seed Extract (preferred brand: NutriBiotic) — 1/4 tsp.
Aubrey Organics® Lemon Blossom Body Splash — 1 Tbsp. (optional)

HOW TO DO IT:

Place Tofu Essential Fatty Acid Cream Base (Formula #1) into a mixing bowl. Chop the aloe vera fillet into small pieces and stir into mixture with a spoon. (Do not use blender.) Add the Green Kamut®, stirring well (mixture will become a dark green color). Break up any lumps with the edge of the spoon and continue stirring. Add the green clay into mixture and combine. Then add the Rosa Mosqueta®, evening primrose and white camellia oils and continue stirring. Add the grapefruit seed extract and the Lemon Blossom Body Splash (optional) last, and stir well into mixture.

HOW TO USE IT:

Use once or twice a week (or more often if needed). After cleansing and toning the skin, apply mask to entire face and leave on for about 10 minutes. Remove mask by gently working a damp washcloth over face, then rinse thoroughly in warm water. Follow with a good, natural moisturizer. IMPORTANT: Keep refrigerated when not in use.

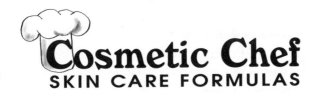

FORMULA #8
Meal & Herbs & Flowers
Facial Scrub for All Skin Types

I **am confident that when you try** this facial scrub, you will be amazed at the results. Most commercial scrubs are formulated with all kinds of synthetic chemicals, and even contain "plastic beads" to help clean the skin. Not this one. This mild exfoliant scrubs away dead skin cells and debris with a gentle sudsing action that's completely natural and easy on your complexion. You can actually feel the tiny grains and herbals working to clear and purify your skin and leave it smooth and lightly moisturized.

INGREDIENTS:
Natural Liquid Soap (preferred brand: Dr. Bronner's Castile Soap) — 1 cup
Psyllium Husks Powder (preferred brand: Yerba Prima) — 1 Tbsp.
Aloe Vera Gel (preferred brand: Aubrey Organics®, or fresh gel from aloe plant
    — just remove fillet from leaf and liquefy in blender) — 2 Tbsp.
Erewhon Organic Brown Rice Cream — 2 Tbsp.
Almond Meal (available in bulk at health food stores) — 1 Tbsp.
Organic Quick Oats (American Prairie) — 1 Tbsp.
Peppermint Leaves — 3 Tbsp.
Wheat Germ — 2 Tbsp.
Aubrey Organics® Lemon Blossom Body Splash (optional) — 1 Tbsp.
Grapefruit Seed Extract (preferred brand: NutriBiotic) — 1 tsp.

HOW TO DO IT:
Place all the dry ingredients in a blender (psyllium husks, almond meal, oats, peppermint leaves and wheat germ) and blend until powder-thin. Add the Natural Liquid Soap, aloe vera gel, the rice cream, the Lemon Blossom (optional) and the grapefruit seed extract, mixing by hand with a spatula until combined. The finished product should be thick, with the consistency of a mask.

HOW TO USE IT:

After cleaning and toning skin, apply mask/scrub to entire face and allow to stay on for 5 to 10 minutes. Splash a small amount of water on your face and work gently over skin with fingers or washcloth, massaging lightly. Rinse thoroughly with warm water, and follow with a natural moisturizer. IMPORTANT: Keep refrigerated when not in use.

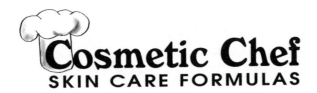

Cosmetic Chef
SKIN CARE FORMULAS

FORMULA #9
Green Cereal Exfoliation Scrub
For Normal to Oily Skin

I have made many exfoliating and skin-regenerating masks and scrubs, but this one is quite special. It uses actual cereal grains and corn meal for their scrubbing and skin-clearing action, and leaves the complexion smooth, with no oily feel. Forget all those scrubs at you local cosmetic counter—totally natural is always best. You will be making and using this one time and again.

INGREDIENTS:

Silken Style Tofu (preferred brand: Nasoya Silken) — 1 cup
Corn Meal (any health food store brand) — 3 Tbsp.
5-Grain Cereal (preferred brand: American Prairie) — 1/3 cup
Lavender Castile Soap (preferred brand: Dr. Bronner's) — 3 Tbsp.
Erewhon Organic Brown Rice Cream — 3 Tbsp.
Lavender Oil (preferred brand: Tisserand) — 16 drops
Grapefruit Seed Extract (preferred brand: NutriBiotic) — 1/2 tsp.
Liquid Vitamin C (preferred brand: TwinLab) — 1/2 tsp.
ProGreens (NutriCology) — 1 tsp.
Vegetable Protein (preferred brand: Naturade) — 1 Tbsp.

HOW TO DO IT:

Drain tofu and place it into a mixing bowl. Next add the various ingredients in the order shown, stirring with a hand mixer or in a blender until uniform.

HOW TO USE IT:

This mask/scrub is great for all skin types, but it is especially effective on aging skin. Its scrubbing and exfoliating action comes from the cereal grains—

they do a gentle job and help get rid of dead skin cells and clear the complexion. Apply mask to face (making sure not to get near or into the eyes) and allow it to stay on for 5 to 10 minutes. Wipe mask off with a warm, damp washcloth and a gentle scrubbing motion, or simply splash your face with water (making sure to keep eyes closed) and work the scrub over the skin with your fingers. Rinse thoroughly in warm water. IMPORTANT: Keep refrigerated when not in use.

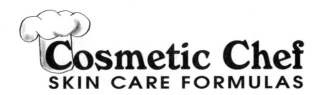

Cosmetic Chef
SKIN CARE FORMULAS

FORMULA #10
The Red Mask
Alpha-Hydroxy Fruit Acid Treatment

O nce you see how this mask looks and smells, you'll want to pour it over a steaming bowl of pasta. Don't. Like our previous guacamole-looking formula, it won't do much for your taste buds, but it will work wonders on your skin. Natural fruit acids from tomatoes and bilberry extract—some of the best exfoliants around—will help slough off drab, dead skin cells to reveal healthy, vibrant skin underneath. And unlike most commercial alpha-hydroxy products, its action is all natural and nonirritating to the skin. I use my rich Tofu Essential Fatty Acid Cream Base to increase absorption and soften and moisturize the complexion.

INGREDIENTS:
Tofu Essential Fatty Acid Cream Base (see Formula #1) — 1/2 cup
Aloe Vera Fillet (preferred brand: Aubrey Organics® Out of the Leaf Aloe Vera
    Fillet, or use fresh fillet from your own aloe plant) — 1 fillet
Organic Tomato Paste (preferred brand: Muir Glen) — 1/4 cup
Bilberry Herb Extract (preferred brands: Frontier, Gaia) — 2 tsp.
Blue Camomile Essential Oil (preferred brand: Aroma Vera) — 2 drops
Grapefruit Seed Extract (preferred brand: NutriBiotic) — 1/4 tsp.
Natural Grain Alcohol — 1/4 cup

HOW TO DO IT:
Place Tofu Essential Fatty Acid Cream Base (Formula #1) into a blender. Add the aloe vera fillet and blend well into mixture. Add the tomato paste and continue blending. Next add the bilberry, the blue camomile oil (only 2 drops), the grapefruit seed extract and the grain alcohol, in that order, and continue mixing in blender until you get a smooth, rich paste.

HOW TO USE IT:

After cleansing and toning your skin, apply mask to face and allow to remain on for about 10 minutes. Splash water on face and wipe mask off with a damp washcloth. You can use this mask once a week, or more often if needed. It will leave your complexion incredibly soft and smooth. IMPORTANT: Keep refrigerated when not in use.

Skin Care Products

Moisturizers, Hydrators & Antiwrinkle Treatments

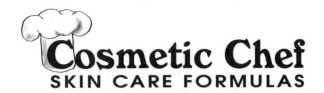

Cosmetic Chef
SKIN CARE FORMULAS

FORMULA #11
Green Tea Daily Moisturizer
For Dry or Mature Skin

Antiwrinkle creams and moisturizers of this type bring in huge sums of money, because nobody is ever completely satisfied with how their skin looks, and almost everyone begins to show some signs of aging after they hit their 30s. The problem with so-called wrinkle-removing moisturizers is that they simply don't work. Their main ingredient, as you probably already know, is mineral oil, a heavy petrochemical that may be just about the worst ingredient you can use on your skin.

Our natural formula uses a high amount of aloe vera gel (organic is best), a wonderful skin hydrator and healing agent. Combined with Rosa Mosqueta® and white camellia oils, two superb emollients, it actually reduces the appearance of fine lines and wrinkles and leaves skin soft and supple.

However, the most important herbal used in this formula is green tea, an excellent skin care ingredient that has been getting a lot of press lately for its strong antioxidant properties. Antioxidants, as we discussed earlier, protect the skin from free radical damage and help prevent certain forms of cancer caused by UV ray exposure and pollution. Alan H. Conway, Ph.D., cancer research specialist at Rutgers State University of New Jersey's College of Pharmacy states: "We do not yet understand the exact mechanisms by which green tea inhibits UVB-induced carcinogenesis, but it may be related to the antioxidant and free radical-scavenging activities of the tea."

This terrific daytime moisturizer is light enough to wear under makeup. Most people see a remarkable improvement in their skin after just a few applications.

INGREDIENTS:
Tofu (soft, preferred brands: Mori-Nu, VitaSoy, Eden Foods) — 1 package (10.5 oz.)
Aloe Vera Gel (preferred brand: Aubrey Organics®, or fresh gel from aloe plant
— just remove fillet from leaf and liquefy in blender) — 4 Tbsp.

Shea Butter (preferred brands: Frontier, Karite-One) — 3 Tbsp.
White Camellia Oil (preferred brand: Aubrey Organics®) — 1 tsp.
Rosa Mosqueta® Rose Hip Seed Oil (available only from Aubrey Organics®) —
    1 tsp.
Jojoba Oil (preferred brand: Aubrey Organics®) — 1 tsp.
Evening Primrose Oil (preferred brand: Aubrey Organics®) — 1 tsp
Flaxseed Oil (preferred brands: Barleans, Arrowhead Mills) — 1 tsp.
Green Tea (Sencha) (preferred brand: Haiku Green Tea) — 2 tea bags
Grapefruit Seed Extract (preferred brand: NutriBiotic) — 1/4 tsp.
St. John's Wort Flower Buds (preferred brand: Gaia) — 1 tsp.
Milk Thistle Seed Extract (preferred brand: Gaia) — 1 tsp.
Lavender Oil (preferred brand: Aura Cacia) — 16 drops.

HOW TO DO IT:

Place the aloe vera, white camellia, Rosa Mosqueta®, jojoba and evening primrose oils into a small, clean sauce pan. Add the St. John's wort flower buds, the shea butter and the milk thistle and grapefruit seed extracts. Place the green tea bags into the oils and heat mixture. As the shea butter melts and mixes with the oils, press the tea bags with a spoon to get the green tea to combine with hot oils. When shea butter is completely melted and mixture is just about to boil, turn off heat and allow to cool. Press tea bags again with a spoon to get all the tea extract into oils. (The color should be a clear, yellowish-green.) Next place the package of tofu into a blender and pour mixture from sauce pan in. Blend until creamy and smooth, then add the flaxseed oil and the lavender oil. Continue mixing in blender until creamy. Place in a bottle or jar and keep cool until ready to use.

HOW TO USE IT:

After cleansing and toning, apply moisturizer to skin and massage gently, concentrating on extra dry or wrinkled areas of the face. This is a rich moisturizer, and a little goes a long way. It makes an excellent night cream, but may also be used as a day cream. Wear it under (or instead of) makeup to help reduce UV ray damage from sun exposure and keep skin hydrated all day long. IMPORTANT: Store in refrigerator when not in use.

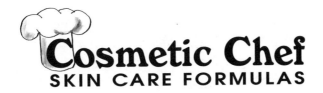

Cosmetic Chef
SKIN CARE FORMULAS

FORMULA #12
Janine's Night & Day Cream
(SPF 15)

I **first made Janine's Night & Day Cream** with Janine Sharell on CNN's *For Women Only* TV show in New York. Janine is from California and had shopped at Mrs. Gooch's health food stores there for years. She asked me to whip up a moisturizer that's every bit as good as one you could buy in a department store, and I did. Janine made it along with me, and later she had to agree—this one is all-natural, and better than anything you can buy at any cosmetic counter.

INGREDIENTS:

Tofu Essential Fatty Acid Cream Base (Formula #1) — 1 cup

Aloe Vera Gel (preferred brand: Aubrey Organics®, or fresh gel from aloe plant — just remove fillet from leaf and liquefy in blender) — 1/2 cup

Rosa Mosqueta® Rose Hip Seed Oil (available only from Aubrey Organics®) — 2 tsp.

White Camellia Oil (preferred brand: Aubrey Organics®) — 2 tsp.

Evening Primrose Oil (preferred brand: Aubrey Organics®) — 2 tsp.

Flaxseed Oil (preferred brands: Barleans, Arrowhead Mills) — 2 tsp.

Jojoba Oil (preferred brand: Aubrey Organics®) — 2 tsp.

Green Kamut® (Green Kamut Corp.) — 2 tsp.

PABA capsules (break open to obtain powder) (preferred brands: Country Life, Solgar) — 1 Tbsp.

Grapefruit Seed Extract (preferred brand: NutriBiotic) — 1/4 tsp.

Aubrey Organics® Angelica Eau de Cologne (optional) — 4 drops

HOW TO DO IT:

Place the Tofu Essential Fatty Acid Cream Base in a clean bowl. Add aloe vera gel, 2 tsp. each of Rosa Mosqueta®, white camellia, evening primrose, flax-seed and jojoba oils one at a time into the cream base, stirring each individual oil well into mixture before moving on to the next one. Then break open PABA capsules and add 1 Tbsp. of powder, stirring well. Add 2 tsp. of the Green Kamut® and continue stirring until green powder is completely blended in, but do not whip up mixture. Finish with the grapefruit seed extract and 4 drops of Angelica Eau de Cologne (the fragrance is optional, but very pleasant). Continue stirring until mixture is uniform, then place into jar and store in the refrigerator.

HOW TO USE IT:

After cleansing and toning the skin, apply a small amount of moisturizer to face and neck and massage gently until it is completely absorbed into the skin.

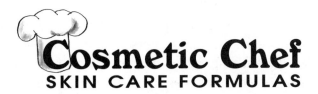

Cosmetic Chef
SKIN CARE FORMULAS

FORMULA #13
Aubrey's Sparkling Mineral Water
Herbal Facial Spray

I was sitting in the lobby of Carnegie Hall waiting for my son, who was rehearsing for a concert there, and in one of the offices they were having a call for ballet dancers. A young dancer sat beside me and put her bag next to my chair. I peeked down inside the bag and saw an extra pair of ballet shoes, a container of yogurt and a bottle of my Sparkling Mineral Water spray.

"Excuse me," I asked, "but could I ask you what you use that for?" She told me it was for her skin. "Want to try it?" she asked, taking it from her bag. Before I had a chance to reply, she pointed the nozzle at me and said, "Close your eyes." She pumped the refreshing fine mist on my face. "What do you think?" she asked. "It's wonderful," I replied. "I never go to a rehearsal without it," she said with a smile.

I was the first cosmetic chemist to make a mineral water spray just for the skin, and it remains one of my favorite products, sold in health food stores all over the world. This special blend of herbs and vitamins in sparkling mineral water not only adds moisture and nutrients to your skin, but is a terrific pick-me-up. Just a "spritz" on the face does wonders to cool and freshen the skin and hydrate the complexion. Make this facial spray and use it during sun exposure, after exercising or any time your skin needs a lift.

INGREDIENTS:

Perrier Sparkling Mineral Water (with lemon, or plain) — 1/2 cup
Aloe Vera Gel (preferred brand: Aubrey Organics®, or fresh gel from aloe plant
    — just remove fillet from leaf and liquefy in blender) — 2 Tbsp.
Milk Thistle (preferred brands: Aura Cacia, Frontier, Gaia) — 2 Tbsp.
Aubrey's Herbal Base (Formula #2) — 7 oz.
Lemon Peel Essential Oil (brands: Aura Cacia, Frontier, Gaia) — 3 drops
Aubrey Organics® Musk Splash (optional) — 3 drops

HOW TO DO IT:

Measure out the Perrier Water and put into a bottle. Add the Herbal Base, aloe vera gel, milk thistle and lemon peel essential oil, then Musk Splash (optional) in that order. Pour mixture into a "fine mist" type pump spray bottle and keep it in the refrigerator when not in use. (This mineral water spray works best on the skin when cool.)

HOW TO USE IT:

Shake well before using. Close your eyes and spray lightly over your face or anywhere your skin needs added moisture. Spray over makeup to set it, and under moisturizers to increase their effectiveness.

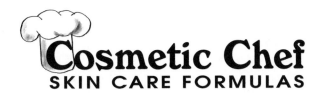

Cosmetic Chef
SKIN CARE FORMULAS

FORMULA #14
Aubrey's Facial Flowers Steam Concentrate
For All Skin Types

I made my first facial steam mixture by combining flowers and herbs. Here's a version of that old formula. The idea is to pour a little of the mixture into a bowl of steaming water and let the steam and herbal blend flow gently over your face for several minutes before you begin your facial. Steaming is excellent therapy for the skin. It soothes and detoxifies the complexion, softens oil deposits and opens to prepare skin for cleansing. This aromatherapy concentrate can also be used in a steamer if you have one.

INGREDIENTS:

Aubrey's Herbal Base (See Formula #2) — l cup
Natural Grain Alcohol — 1/2 cup
Witch Hazel (preferred brand: Dickenson's) — 1/2 cup
Aubrey Organics® Lemon Blossom Body Splash — 1 Tbsp.

HOW TO DO IT:

Pour alcohol and witch hazel into a mixing bowl. Add the Herbal Base (Formula #2). Add the Lemon Blossom Body Splash to the mixture last.

HOW TO USE IT:

When you're giving yourself a complete facial (as described in the skin section of this book), you will definitely want to steam your complexion before cleansing. Shake well before using, then simply put 3 or 4 tablespoons of this concentrate into a bowl of steaming water, place a towel over your head to create a tent, and let the steam flow over your face for 1-2 minutes, keeping your eyes closed. Since this formula contains both alcohol and witch hazel, it will not spoil. You may keep it refrigerated if you wish, although it isn't necessary.

Body Care Products
Soaps & Body Lotions

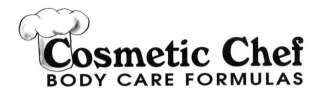

Cosmetic Chef
BODY CARE FORMULAS

FORMULA #15
Lavender Liquid Body Soap
For All Skin Types

You will be using a lot of this body soap. You'll want to keep a bottle of it by every sink, shower or tub in the house because it is very gentle on the skin. It rinses clean, without leaving a soap film or a tight, dry feeling the way most soaps do. Try it and you'll see what we mean.

INGREDIENTS:

Pure Lavender Castile Soap (preferred brand: Dr. Bronner's) — 1 cup
Aubrey Organics® Seasoap — 1/2 cup
Shea Butter (preferred brands: Frontier, Karite-One) — 2 tsp.
Lavender Oil (preferred brand: Tisserand) — 8 drops
Psyllium Husks Powder (preferred brand: Yerba Prima) — 2 Tbsp.
Grapefruit Seed Extract (preferred brand: NutriBiotic) — 1/2 tsp.

HOW TO DO IT:

Pour 1 cup of Dr. Bronner's Lavender Castile Soap into a mixing bowl and add 1/4 cup of Seasoap. Seasoap is thick, so you'll have to scoop it out of the jar and mix it carefully into the castile soap, making sure there are no lumps. (You may be able to use a hand mixer sparingly, just enough to get the Seasoap blended, but do not over-mix, as this will cause formula to foam). Place the shea butter in a sauce pan on the stove and slowly melt it, then add it to the mix. Add the 8 drops of lavender and the psyllium husks powder and stir well into batch. The psyllium husks powder will thicken the product considerably. You must get all this powder blended well into the solution, but using a hand mixer at this point will cause quite a bit of foam. It is possible, with a little patience, to get the powders blended in by manual stirring. Even if the resulting body soap turns out slightly grainy, this will not affect how it works. This is a "high sudsing" cleanser, and very good for your skin. Add the grapefruit seed extract last.

HOW TO USE IT:
This is a soft and gentle body soap, ideal for shower and bath, and great for the entire family. IMPORTANT: Keep refrigerated when not in use.

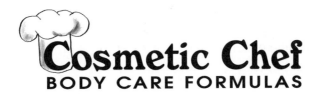

Cosmetic Chef
BODY CARE FORMULAS

FORMULA #16
Evening Primrose Hand & Body Lotion

I introduced the use of evening primrose oil to the cosmetic industry many years ago, and have created lotions, conditioners and shampoos using this very special oil, which is one of the few known sources of gamma-linolenic acid, an essential fatty acid also found in mother's milk. One of the most pleasant effects of this oil is that it leaves the skin smooth and soft, but it is most valued for its soothing and healing properties on itchy, irritated or damaged skin. Evening primrose oil has been used to treat the unpleasant symptoms of topical yeast infections, eczema and other skin conditions. Included in baby products, it helps soothe cradle cap and infantile eczema and control and prevent diaper rash. This superb lotion, similar to the one I've been making at Aubrey Organics® for years, is excellent for all sorts of skin problems, including dryness, flaking and "dish pan hands." (Note: Evening primrose oil works best when included in a formula or otherwise diluted. It should *not* be used full strength.)

INGREDIENTS:
Tofu (silken, soft) (preferred brand: Mori-Nu) — 1 cup
Aloe Vera Fillet (preferred brand: Aubrey Organics® Out of the Leaf, or use the
    fresh gel from the leaf of your own aloe plant) — about 1/2 cup, or 1 fillet.
Evening Primrose Oil (preferred brand: Aubrey Organics®) — 2 Tbsp.
Grapefruit Seed Extract (preferred brand: NutriBiotic) — 1/4 tsp.
Shea Butter (preferred brands: Frontier, Karite-One) — 2 Tbsp.

HOW TO DO IT:
Place ingredients into blender in order shown, then blend just long enough to give the mixture a creamy consistency.

HOW TO USE IT:

This all-purpose hand and body lotion can be used daily on rough, dry hands and on flaking, irritated or sun-damaged areas of the skin. IMPORTANT: Keep refrigerated when not in use.

Hair Care Products

Shampoos, Conditioners & Styling Sprays

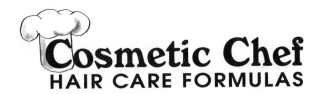

Cosmetic Chef
HAIR CARE FORMULAS

FORMULA #17
Natural Almond Amino Acid Shampoo
For Normal to Oily Hair

S hampoos are slightly difficult to make by hand, but the greater availability of many natural ingredients in health food stores now gives us more flexibility with what we can do at home.

The following shampoo is terrific, and leaves the hair clean, soft and lustrous. When you are watching TV and you see one of those shampoo commercials with a girl swinging her hair around and saying her shampoo is an all-out organic experience, you can have a bit of a laugh. No shampoo you can buy at a cosmetic counter is as natural as this almond shampoo. This formula makes about nine ounces of shampoo.

INGREDIENTS:
Almond Castile Soap (preferred brand: Dr. Bronner's) — 1 cup
Liquid Vitamin C (preferred brand: TwinLab) — 4 drops
Aloe Vera Gel (preferred brand: Aubrey Organics®, or fresh gel from aloe plant —
    just remove fillet from leaf and liquefy in blender) — 2 Tbsp.
Grapefruit Seed Extract (preferred brand: NutriBiotic) — 1/4 tsp.
Max Amino Caps (amino acids with B-6) (preferred brand: Country Life) —
    4 caps.
Biotin (preferred brand: TwinLab) — 1 cap.
Vegetable Glycerine — 1/2 tsp.
Jojoba Oil (preferred brand: Aubrey Organics®) — 1/2 tsp.
Yucca and Burdock Extract (preferred brand: TwinLab) — 1 Tbsp.
Shea Butter (preferred brands: Frontier, Karite-One) — 1 tsp.
Psyllium Husks Powder (preferred brand: Yerba Prima) — 2 Tbsp.

HOW TO DO IT:

Pour 1 cup of Dr. Bronner's Almond Castile Soap into a mixing bowl. Add all ingredients one at a time in the order listed. Using a spatula, slowly stir each ingredient in before moving on to the next one, breaking up any lumps by squeezing them against the side of the mixing bowl with the spatula. (Do not use a blender or electric mixer, as this will create too much suds.) As with the previous formula, the vitamin capsules should be snapped or cut open and the entire contents poured into the mixture. The psyllium husks powder will make the product thicker, but be careful—if the product is too thick it will not be easy to pour into a bottle, so cut back on this ingredient if mixture is getting too dense— a semi-thick shampoo is best. When you're finished, the shampoo will be a light coffee color and will smell slightly of almonds.

HOW TO USE IT:

Shake well before using. Apply your Almond Amino Acid Shampoo like any other shampoo. Rinse thoroughly and do a second lather if needed. All your friends are going to be asking you to make them a bottle as soon as they see how shiny and healthy your hair looks. IMPORTANT: Keep refrigerated when not in use.

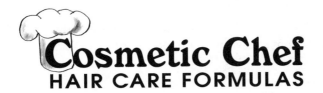

Cosmetic Chef
HAIR CARE FORMULAS

FORMULA #18
Rosa Mosqueta® Super Protein Shampoo

This shampoo is excellent for dull, damaged hair, but all hair types will benefit from this ultra-nourishing formula. Protein is one of the best nutrients you can put on your hair, and liquid collagen protein is easily absorbed and goes to work instantly to give the hair body and strength and help repair split ends. Rosa Mosqueta® and lavender oils, two superb emollients, help heal and condition the hair shaft, and aloe vera soothes the scalp and adds moisture. I've been making this type of shampoo for more than ten years and get nothing but praise for the way it makes the hair look and feel.

INGREDIENTS:

Aubrey Organics® Seasoap — 1 cup
Aloe Vera Gel (preferred brand: Aubrey Organics®, or fresh gel from aloe plant
    — just remove fillet from leaf and liquefy in blender) — 1/4 cup
Collagen Liquid Protein (preferred brand: TwinLab) — 1 tsp.
Rosa Mosqueta® Rose Hip Seed Oil (available only from Aubrey Organics®) —
    1 tsp.
Lavender Oil (preferred brand: Gaia Herbs) — 1/2 tsp.
Grapefruit Seed Extract (preferred brand: NutriBiotic) — 1 tsp.

HOW TO DO IT:

Scoop Seasoap out of jar and into a mixing bowl. Add the other ingredients one at a time in order listed. Using a spatula, stir each carefully into mixture before moving on to the next one. (Do not use a blender, as this will create too much suds.) Pour mixture into a bottle and store in refrigerator until you're ready to use it.

HOW TO USE IT:

Shake well before using. Apply to hair as you would any shampoo, lather, then rinse thoroughly. Repeat if needed, then follow with a good conditioner. This makes an excellent everyday shampoo for all hair types. (Note: This is not a vegan product.)

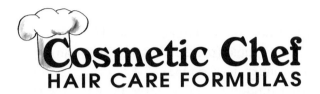

Cosmetic Chef
HAIR CARE FORMULAS

FORMULA #19
Dr. Duke's Hair Saver
Rosemary & Sage Shampoo

Dr. James Duke, the noted herbalist, has been telling me for years that I should make a Rosemary & Sage Shampoo to go with my Rosemary & Sage Hair Rinse. (You can make your own Rosemary & Sage Hair Rinse with 4 parts of rosemary oil and 4 parts of sage oil in 16 parts of witch hazel. The ingredients will separate in the bottle, so you'll have to shake the bottle well each time before using it.) Dr. Duke holds forth on the great hair care values of rosemary, sage, comfrey and other herbals for hair loss and dandruff in *The Green Pharmacy* (Rodale Press, 1997), as useful a reference book as you'll ever find. As we mentioned earlier, in *Hamlet*, Shakespeare has Ophelia say, "Here's rosemary. That's for remembrance." Perhaps the Bard of Avon was onto something, because Dr. Duke says perhaps rosemary is a "brain saver" (anti-Alzheimer ingredient) as well as a hair saver, but you can learn more about that from Dr. Duke. We give you Rosemary & Sage Shampoo for what's on top of your head rather than what's inside. I've come up with a natural shampoo you can make using these and other great herbs, and I've named it after Dr. Duke. Here is the formula:

INGREDIENTS:

Peppermint Castile Soap (preferred brand: Dr. Bronner's) — 1 cup
Liquid Vitamin C (preferred brand: TwinLab) — 4 drops
Aloe Vera Gel (preferred brand: Aubrey Organics®, or fresh gel from aloe plant
    — just remove fillet from leaf and liquefy in blender) — 2 Tbsp.
Grapefruit Seed Extract (preferred brand: NutriBiotic) — 1/4 tsp.
Max Amino Caps (amino acids with B-6) (brand: Country Life) — 4 caps.

Sage Oil (brands: Aura Cacia, Frontier, Gaia) — 1 tsp.
Rosemary Oil (brands: Aura Cacia, Frontier, Gaia) — 1 tsp.

181

Comfrey Root Extract (brands: Aura Cacia, Frontier, Gaia) — 1 tsp.
Biotin (600 mcg.) (preferred brand: TwinLab) — 2 caps.
Vegetable Glycerine — 1/2 tsp.
Jojoba Oil (preferred brand: Aubrey Organics®) — 1/2 tsp.
Yucca and Burdock Root Liquid (preferred brand: TwinLab) — 1 Tbsp.
Shea Butter (brands: Frontier, Karite-One) — 1 tsp.
Psyllium Husks Powder (preferred brand: Yerba Prima) — 2 Tbsp.

HOW TO DO IT:

Pour in 1 cup of Dr. Bronner's Peppermint Castile Soap into a mixing bowl. Add all ingredients one at a time in the order listed. Using a spatula, slowly stir in the ingredients. (Do not use a blender or electric mixer, as this will create too much suds.) Break up any lumps by squeezing them against the sides of the mixing bowl with the spatula, and continue stirring mixture slowly. (The vitamin capsules should be snapped or cut open and their entire contents poured into the mixture.) The psyllium husks powder will make the product thicker, but cut back on this ingredient if mixture is getting too dense—a semi-thick shampoo is best. When you're finished, the shampoo will be a light coffee color and have a mild, pleasant fragrance.

HOW TO USE:

Shake well before using. Use it daily and make your Rosemary & Sage Hair Rinse to go with it. Shampoo as usual, and follow with the rinse. If your hair is dry, you'll want to finish off with a cream-based conditioner.

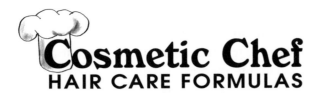

Cosmetic Chef
HAIR CARE FORMULAS

FORMULA #20
Blue Green Algae Hair Rescue Shampoo
For Problem Scalp

I first made a blue green algae shampoo in 1997 as a companion to my blue green algae hair mask (see Formula# 21). Blue green algae is one of the best sources of vegetable protein and is also high in amino acids, vitamins and minerals. This nourishing formula is recommended for all types of hair, and works particularly well on problem scalp and dandruff. Use the shampoo and hair mask together for best results. Your hair will thank you.

INGREDIENTS:

Aubrey Organics® Herbal Liquid Body Soap — 1 cup
Blue Green Algae Powder (preferred brand: Klamath) — 1 Tbsp.
Tea Tree Oil (preferred brand: Desert Essence) — 6 drops
Pine Essential Oil (preferred brand: Tisserand) — 1/2 tsp.
Grapefruit Seed Extract (preferred brand: NutriBiotic) — 1 tsp.
Max Amino Caps (amino acids with B-6, preferred brand: Country Life) —
    1 cap.
L-Cysteine (500 mg.) (preferred brand: Country Life) — 1 cap.
Aloe Vera Gel (preferred brand: Aubrey Organics®, or fresh gel from aloe plant
    — just remove fillet from leaf and liquify in blender) — 1 Tbsp.
Shea Butter (preferred brands: Frontier, Karite-One) — 1 tsp.

HOW TO DO IT:

In a clean mixing bowl combine the blue green algae powder and the soap a little bit at a time, carefully stirring them together. If you have trouble getting them to mix well, use an electric hand mixer on slow speed just long enough to blend, but don't over-mix, as this will create too much suds. Put in the 6 drops of tea tree oil and continue mixing with a spatula. Stir in the 1/2 teaspoon of pine oil and mix well, then add the grapefruit seed extract. (You may notice the mixture thins out a little at this point—this is a natural reaction.) Next break open the Max Amino Caps and L-cysteine caps and add the powder, carefully blending each in. Finish your shampoo formula by adding the aloe vera and shea butter. (To add the shea butter, dip out a little more than a teaspoonful and heat in a pan just until it melts [do not boil], then add to mixture, stirring in slowly with the spatula.) Pour your Blue Green Algae Hair Rescue Shampoo into a bottle and run to the shower or bath to try it out!

HOW TO USE IT:

This shampoo is part of your two-step hair care plan for scalp problems and dry, brittle or salon-damaged hair. First apply the Blue Green Algae Hair Rescue Mask (Formula #21 on next page) to your hair and let it do its work for about 15 minutes or so; then wash it out with the shampoo. Use both regularly to help control dandruff and other scalp problems and give your hair body and shine. You'll be able to wear dark suits again and will see all sorts of scalp problems start to clear up in a couple of weeks. IMPORTANT: Keep refrigerated when not in use.

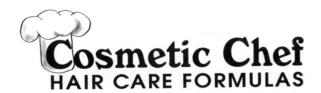

Cosmetic Chef
HAIR CARE FORMULAS

FORMULA #21
Blue Green Algae Hair Rescue Mask
Natural Treatment for Problem Hair and Scalp

T he **"Green Hair Mask,"** as it came to be known at seminars, was designed to work together with the Blue Green Algae Hair Rescue Shampoo, but it also works very well on its own. I first made it at a health food seminar in Orlando, FL, where nearly one thousand people got to try it out. The next day our phone was ringing off the hook! "This conditioner really works!" I kept hearing over and over. It does. Most people use the hair mask once or twice a week, and the Blue Green Algae Shampoo daily. Here's how to make the mask:

INGREDIENTS:

Tofu (silken, soft) (preferred brand: Mori-Nu) — 1 cup
Blue Green Algae (preferred brand: Klamath) — 1 Tbsp.
Max Amino Caps (amino acids with B-6) (preferred brand: Country Life) —
    4 caps.
Biotin (600 mcg.) (preferred brand: TwinLab) — 1 cap.
L-Cysteine (500 mg.) (preferred brand: Country Life) — 1 cap.
ProGreens® Powder (NutriCology) — 1 tsp.
Horsetail Grass (alcohol-free) (preferred brand: Nature's Answer) — 1/2 tsp.
Sage Oil (preferred brands: Aura Cacia, Gaia) — 1/4 tsp.
Rosemary Oil (preferred brands: Aura Cacia, Gaia) — 1/4 tsp.
Comfrey Extract (preferred brand: Herbs of Light) — 1/4 tsp.
Rosewater (preferred brand: Frontier) — 1 Tbsp.
Vegetable Glycerine — 1 Tbsp.
Lavender Oil (preferred brand: Gaia) — 1/2 tsp.
Natural Grain Alcohol (150 proof) — 1 Tbsp.
Grapefruit Seed Extract (preferred brand: NutriBiotic) — 2 tsp.

Shea Butter (preferred brands: Frontier, Karite-One) — 1 Tbsp.
Tea Tree Oil (preferred brand: Desert Essence) — 1 drop only

HOW TO DO IT:

Place tofu into the mixing bowl, add the blue green algae, and using a hand mixer, blend together until mixture is a smooth, dark green. (Though the actual mixture may be slightly grainy, this doesn't matter.) Cut or snap open the Max Amino Caps, biotin and L-cysteine caps and blend in. Be sure to get all the vitamin powder into mixture, stirring each carefully for a few seconds. Add the rest of the ingredients, except for the shea butter, in order shown. In a small sauce pan, melt shea butter on the stove until soft, then blend into mixture.

HOW TO USE IT:

When you're finished you will have a dark, blue-green mask. It works best when applied while the hair is dry. Work it well into ends of the hair and into scalp, then leave it on for 15 minutes. Let it go to work, then shampoo out and rinse thoroughly.

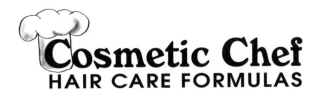

Cosmetic Chef
HAIR CARE FORMULAS

FORMULA #22
Jojoba & Aloe Instant Hair Conditioning Cream

T his may seem like the simplest formula in this book, but it makes a superb "instant" hair conditioner. I created it a long time ago and improved on it through the years. This rich conditioner is excellent for dull, dry, over-processed or chemically damaged hair. You'll get rave reviews.

INGREDIENTS:

Tofu (silken, soft) (preferred brand: Mori-Nu) — 1 cup
Aloe Vera Fillets (preferred brand: Aubrey Organics® Out of the Leaf, or use the fresh fillet from your own aloe plant) — 1 cup
Jojoba Oil (preferred brand: Aubrey Organics®) — 1 Tbsp.
Grapefruit Seed Extract (preferred brand: NutriBiotic)—1/4 tsp.
Max Amino Caps (amino acids with B-6) (preferred brand: Country Life) — 4 caps.
Shea Butter (preferred brands: Frontier, Karite-One) — 2 Tbsp.
Carrot Juice — 1 Tbsp.

HOW TO DO IT:

Place the tofu, aloe vera fillets and jojoba oil in a blender, then blend ingredients until they have a smooth, creamy consistency. Add the grapefruit seed extract, then pour in the Max Amino Caps by opening capsules and dumping the powder into your mixture. Next add the shea butter (you don't need to melt it— just combine it into the mixture with the blender). Add the carrot juice last and mix into batch. The resulting mixture should be smooth, and yellow in color.

HOW TO USE IT:

Simply work this instant hair conditioner through your hair, concentrating on the ends. Allow a couple of minutes for it to do its work, then rinse thoroughly.

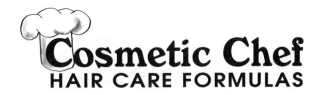

Cosmetic Chef
HAIR CARE FORMULAS

FORMULA #23
Tangle-Go Luster Spray

Tangle-Go is a product I've made for years. It not only gives the hair a beautiful luster, but helps the brush or comb "glide" through it without a snarl or tangle—hence its name. You make it almost the same way you make the hairspray on the following page, except the idea of this spray is not to "hold" the hair but to condition it and give it sheen. Luster sprays like this one are often made with lanolin, but this is a more effective formula, containing white camellia and evening primrose oils, excellent emollients that add moisture and shine without leaving a greasy feel on the hair.

INGREDIENTS:

Natural Grain Alcohol (150 proof) — 4 oz.
Vegetable Glycerine — 2 Tbsp.
Evening Primrose Oil (preferred brand: Aubrey Organics®) — 1 tsp.
White Camellia Oil (preferred brand: Aubrey Organics®) — 1/2 tsp.
Lavender Essential Oil (preferred brands: Tisserand, Gaia Herbs) — 3 drops

HOW TO DO IT:

Measure out the alcohol, pour it into a clean container and set aside. In a separate container, place the glycerine, evening primrose, white camellia and lavender oils together and mix. Pour the glycerin-oil mixture into the alcohol and mix together until uniform.

HOW TO USE IT:

Pour your Tangle-Go Luster Spray into a pump bottle with a fine-mist spray action. Shake well before using to make sure mixture is uniform, then spray on damp hair after shampooing, and in-between shampoos to add softness, manageability and shine.

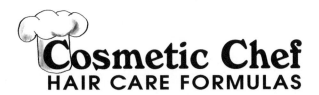

Cosmetic Chef
HAIR CARE FORMULAS

FORMULA #24
White Camellia Amino Acid Hairspray
Regular Hold and Super Hold Formulas

Hairsprays are awful—let's face it! All drug store brands reek of cheap, synthetic perfumes. But worse, most commercial formulas use plastics such as PVP to coat your hair and make it stiff and brittle. And the aerosol cans many of them come in aren't doing the environment any good. Years ago I set out to create an all-natural hairspray made with herbal gums that would rival anybody's "ultra-hold" formula. Gum arabic is a far superior ingredient to plastic and other harsh synthetics, and it won't build up on your hair, dry it out or cause flaking. The trick to making this hairspray is to strain it well so that it will not clog the spray unit.

Regular Hold Formula:

INGREDIENTS:
Natural Grain Alcohol — 4 oz.
Gum Arabic (Acacia) (preferred brand: Delamo Chemicals "spray dried" acacia) — 2 tsp.
Vegetable Glycerine — 1/2 tsp.
White Camellia Oil (preferred brand: Aubrey Organics®) — 1/8 tsp.
Max Amino Caps (amino acids with B-6) (preferred brand: Country Life) — 1/8 tsp. (one capsule)
Lavender Essential Oil (preferred brands: Tisserand, Gaia) — 4 drops

HOW TO DO IT:
Measure out the alcohol and pour it into a blender. Add the gum arabic, then open Max Amino Cap, pour in the powder and blend at high speed. Immediately after mixing, strain liquid through a paper towel into a clean container.

191

(You don't want any "floaters" in the liquid.) In a separate container, place the glycerine and the white camellia oil, and stir. Pour this mixture into the alcohol-gum-amino acid mixture and continue stirring. If needed, use blender again to combine.

Pour hairspray into a spray bottle with a "fine mist" nozzle. If you can't find one, you can always buy a cheap hairspray in a pump bottle, pour the contents down the drain, clean it out well, and put your own herbal hairspray in it.

HOW TO USE IT:

Shake well before using. Spray on the hair just as you would any hairspray to add natural body and a "soft hold" to your hair. The Super Hold formula below will give you even more hold and body. (Note: Be sure not to get hairspray in your eyes. It contains alcohol and will burn. Also, it is flammable, so don't use it near an open flame.)

Super Hold Formula:

By mixing more gum arabic, you will create a hairspray with a stronger hold. You can start with 4 teaspoons, and could probably go as high as 8 teaspoons of gum arabic, but bear in mind that you will have to strain this mixture through a paper towel two or three times before placing it in a spray bottle, as the heavier formula is more likely to clog the sprayer.

Special Formulas

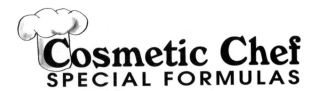

Cosmetic Chef
SPECIAL FORMULAS

FORMULA #25
"Away with You"
Herbal Insect Deterrent Spray

This is by far the finest insect repellent spray anywhere, at any price. You can use it to keep all sorts of insects from even landing on your skin. It isn't greasy at all, and it doesn't have that awful "petrochemical" smell. But the most important thing is that this natural formula contains nothing toxic—no synthetic pesticides or chemicals of any kind. And it's so gentle, you can spray it on the most sensitive skin.

When I first made it, I gave it a tough trial. I went deep into a Florida swamp, sprayed some on and climbed into my kayak. To be fair about the test, I sprayed it on one arm, but not on the other. You can guess what happened. I had many bites on the unsprayed arm, but none on the arm sprayed with "Away with You!" Then I set out to see if this formula could offer protection from another kind of Florida pest—a type of insect so small, their common name is "no-see-'ums." They are around in the daytime, but come out in force at night, and are so tiny they can go right through a screen. I put on the spray, took my dog for a walk and sat outdoors for a long time. No bites! You're going to love this spray, and you'll be delighted with how great it smells without one drop of perfume oil. The magic is in the mixture of the herbs.

INGREDIENTS:

Vegetable Glycerine — 1 tsp.
Liquid Lecithin (preferred brand: Country Life) — 1/4 tsp.
Soybean Oil (preferred brand: Spectrum Naturals) — 1 tsp.
Lavender Oil (preferred brand: Tisserand) — 8 drops
Rosemary Oil (preferred brands: Aura Cacia, Frontier, Gaia) — 1 drop
Sage Oil (preferred brands: Aura Cacia, Frontier, Gaia) — 1 drop
Natural Grain Alcohol — 1/2 cup

HOW TO DO IT:

In a mixing bowl, add ingredients one at a time in the order shown, stirring each well into the mixture before moving on to the next. Measure out the alcohol last and add it slowly to the combined oils, then mix in a blender.

HOW TO USE IT:

Pour your mixture into a pump spray bottle that has a "fine" spray pattern. Next write these instructions on the bottle: Shake Well Before Using. Do Not Spray Near Eyes. When going to the beach, or anywhere outside during the summer months (or any time insects are out), spray all exposed areas of the body. You will be delighted with the results. No bites! IMPORTANT: Keep refrigerated when not in use.

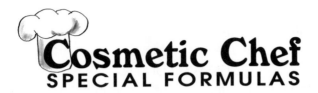

Cosmetic Chef
SPECIAL FORMULAS

FORMULA #26
Kava Kava Relaxing Bath Emulsion

The first product I ever made, back in 1967, was called Relax-R-Bath. Before then, I used to make it at home for my own use, and on cold, chill-in-the-bones New York nights, I'd put some into a hot tub, then lay back and let it do its job. The key ingredient in this wonderful bath elixir is powdered ginger root. Relax-R-Bath is so popular all over the world, that it has remained on my best seller list all this time—over three decades! That's quite a record!

I have since formulated other very successful bath products, including Eucalyptus Spa Bath, with cooling eucalyptus oil, and NSB (Natural Sports Bath), a soothing bath oil for athletes and other active people. I've combined elements of all my herbal bath products into this formula you can make in your own kitchen. It contains kava kava, a natural analgesic that relieves sore muscles and actually helps them relax. Just remember, once the word gets out, people might start dropping by your house at all hours to take a bath!

INGREDIENTS:
Aubrey Organics® Herbal Liquid Body Soap — 1 cup
Ginger Root Extract (preferred brands: Aura Cacia, Frontier, Gaia) —
    2 Tbsp.
Peppermint Oil (preferred brands: Aura Cacia, Frontier, Gaia)— 1/4 tsp.
Eucalyptus Oil (preferred brands: Aura Cacia, Frontier, Gaia) — 1/4 tsp.
Rosemary Oil (preferred brands: Aura Cacia, Frontier, Gaia) — 1/4 tsp.
Orange Blossom Oil (preferred brand: Tisserand) — 1/4 tsp.
Lavender Oil (preferred brand: Tisserand) — 1/4 tsp.
Cypress Oil (preferred brand: Tisserand) — 1/4 tsp.
Cedar Wood Oil (preferred brand: Tisserand) — 1/4 tsp.

Pine Oil (preferred brands: Aura Cacia, Frontier, Gaia) — 1/4 tsp.
Lemon Oil (preferred brand: Herbs of Light) — 1 tsp.
Kava Kava (preferred brands: Gaia, Pioneer) — 2 Tbsp.
Natural Grain Alcohol — 1 cup

HOW TO DO IT:

To begin, combine the essential oils of peppermint, eucalyptus, rosemary, orange blossom, lavender, cypress, cedar wood, pine and lemon into a bottle or jar with a tight-fitting lid. This is your essential oil stock for making the bath emulsion. Then, into a clean mixing bowl, pour the Herbal Liquid Body Soap, add exactly 1 tablespoon of the essential oils mixture you've just prepared, and stir well together. (Set rest of essential oil mixture aside and keep refrigerated until next time.) Then add the ginger root oil to your bath emulsion mixture. Do not whip up or stir in a blender, but simply hand-stir the ingredients together with a spatula until uniform. Add the alcohol and the kava kava. Now you're ready for your bath.

HOW TO USE IT:

Shake well before using. This is the most relaxing bath oil you'll experience. I guarantee it will leave the most uptight person as mellow and supple as melting butter. Put about 1 ounce of mixture into a tub of hot water (as hot as you can stand), then step into the tub and relax. Share your mixture with friends, but be sure to always keep some on hand for your own use! By the way, when you're coming down with a cold or the flu, try soaking for several minutes in one of these baths. Then drink a cup of echinacea and goldenseal tea and go to bed. The next morning you'll probably feel much better.

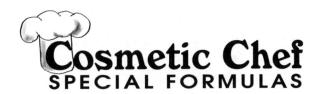

Cosmetic Chef
SPECIAL FORMULAS

FORMULA #27
"Yeast-Away"
Anti-Yeast & Itch Prevention Cream

C*andida albicans* **is a problem** that affects thousands of men and women. The catch phrase for this condition is "yeast infection," which often shows up on the skin, particularly under the arms and in the groin area. One of the best natural treatments for candida is *acidophilus,* which can be obtained as a supplement in the refrigerated section of your health food store, and is also found in yogurt.

In the 1970s I wrote about tea tree oil, an herbal oil that has been shown to reduce and/or eliminate the itching and discomfort of candida when used topically. I've since created an anti-itch product using tea tree oil combined with oregano oil, another superb antibacterial; however my Aubrey Organics® formula is slightly different. The formula below uses organic yogurt as its carrying agent, which means you'll need to make fresh batches frequently. Try this special lotion and say good-bye to itchy nights and days.

INGREDIENTS:
Organic Yogurt (with active *acidophilus* cultures) (preferred brand: Stonyfield Farm) — 8 oz.
Oregano Oil (preferred brand: North American Herb & Spice) — 6 Tbsp.
Peppermint Oil (preferred brands: Aura Cacia, Frontier, Gaia) — 7 drops
Eucalyptus Oil (preferred brands: Aura Cacia, Frontier, Gaia) — 28 drops
Tea Tree Oil (preferred brands: Aura Cacia, Desert Essence) — 28 drops
Camphor Oil (preferred brands: Aura Cacia, Frontier, Gaia) — 7 drops
Grapefruit Seed Extract (preferred brand: NutriBiotic) — 1/8 tsp.
Evening Primrose Oil (preferred brand: Aubrey Organics®) — 4 tsp.
Natural Grain Alcohol — 5 Tbsp.
Aubrey Organics® Lemon Blossom Body Splash (optional) — 1/4 tsp.

HOW TO DO IT:
Place alcohol into a clean container. Measure ingredients carefully, then com-

bine them one at a time into the alcohol, stirring by hand. Next place the yogurt in a separate container and add the alcohol-oil mixture a little bit at a time, stirring until blended with the yogurt. (You can use a blender, but be sure not to over-mix, as this will cause it to become too thin.) The end result should be a semi-thick-to-thin lotion. The Lemon Blossom Body Splash is optional, but it helps disguise the somewhat unpleasant smell of the tea tree oil. (You may add more Lemon Blossom Body Splash if you wish.)

HOW TO USE IT:

Apply the cream to problem areas of the skin. You may experience a slight "burning" sensation in more sensitive areas, but this will go away shortly. Use the cream two or three times daily, especially at night when itching can be at its worst. Important: Avoid getting cream into eyes. Be sure to wash hands after use. Though the grapefruit seed extract and alcohol help preserve it, you may want to keep this lotion in the refrigerator.

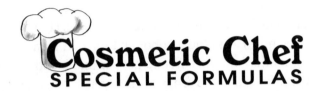

Cosmetic Chef
SPECIAL FORMULAS

FORMULA #28
Feet Rescue
Massage Cream for Troubled Feet

Through the years I have received numerous requests for an all-natural foot cream. Recently, a podiatrist who frequently treats diabetic patients contacted me about creating a formula to increase circulation and help heal dry, cracked feet. I set out to make such a formula. My Feet Relief is now available in health food stores, and Olympic racewalker Debbi Lawrence liked it so much, she endorsed the product and signed the bottle. Here's how to make a similar formula at home.

INGREDIENTS:

Tofu (preferred brand: Mori-Nu "Silken") — 1 package (10.5 oz.)
Aloe Vera Fillet (preferred brand: Aubrey Organics® Out of the Leaf, or use the fresh fillet from your own aloe plant) — 3 Tbsp.
Shea Butter (preferred brands: Frontier, Karite-One) — 1/4 cup
Natural Grain Alcohol — 3 Tbsp.
White Camellia Oil (preferred brand: Aubrey Organics®) — 3 Tbsp.
Cayenne Pepper Oil (preferred brands: Aura Cacia, Frontier) — 2-3 Tbsp.
Eucalyptus Oil (preferred brands: Aura Cacia, Frontier, Gaia) — 3 drops
Ginger Oil (preferred brands: Aura Cacia, Frontier, Gaia) — 2 drops
Peppermint Oil (preferred brands: Aura Cacia, Frontier, Gaia) — 2 drops
Tea Tree Oil (preferred brands: Aura Cacia, Desert Essence) — 2 drops
Camphor Oil (preferred brands: Aura Cacia, Frontier, Gaia) — 2 drops
Wintergreen Oil (preferred brands: Aura Cacia, Frontier, Gaia) — 2 drops
Grapefruit Seed Extract (preferred brand: NutriBiotic) — 1/2 tsp.

HOW TO DO IT:

Drain tofu and break up into pieces. Place pieces into a blender, add the aloe vera fillet and the shea butter (no need to melt shea butter). Turn on blender and let it mix for a minute, then turn off, move the ingredients around by hand, and turn on blender again. Do this until the mixture is uniform. (It may be a bit lumpy at first, but don't over-mix.) Add the alcohol and turn on blender. The mixture will begin to look smooth. Add the cayenne pepper and blend. Put in the white camellia oil and blend. Then add the drops of eucalyptus, ginger, peppermint, tea tree, camphor and wintergreen oils. Continue blending until it is a smooth cream, then place in a clean jar and keep refrigerated when not in use. This formula makes 11 oz., or about 1 $\frac{2}{3}$ cup.

HOW TO USE IT:

Wash feet in warm water, then apply cream and massage well into the skin. You may want to apply the cream before walking or running to warm up muscles, and after to soothe sore, overworked feet. Keep cream refrigerated when not in use. IMPORTANT: Keep cream away from the eyes, as the cayenne pepper will cause intense burning. Always wash your hands after each use. Do not apply cream to broken skin.

Baby Care Products

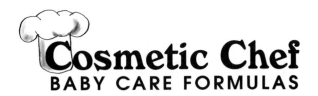

Cosmetic Chef
BABY CARE FORMULAS

FORMULA #29
Natural Baby's Evening Primrose Shampoo

We are all familiar with so-called "no more tears" baby shampoos. These formulas do not keep detergents and other harsh ingredients from harming the eyes—they simply block your baby's ability to *feel* the burning. They also interfere with the eye's tearing mechanism, which is nature's way of washing out the irritating substance. Stay away from "no more tears" formulas—in the long run, they do much more harm than good. Instead, try this ultra-mild shampoo made with herbs and vitamins. It will leave baby's hair soft and clean, and its healing formula, rich in evening primrose oil, has been shown to help clear up infantile eczema, "cradle cap" and other scalp problems.

INGREDIENTS:
Aubrey Organics® Seasoap — 1 cup
Aloe Vera Gel (preferred brand: Aubrey Organics®, or fresh gel from aloe plant
   — just remove fillet from leaf and liquefy in blender) — 1/4 cup
Collagen Liquid Protein (preferred brand: Twin Labs) — 1 tsp.
Evening Primrose Oil (preferred brand: Aubrey Organics®) — 2 tsp.
Lavender Oil (preferred brands: Aura Cacia, Frontier, Gaia) — 1/2 tsp.
Grapefruit Seed Extract (preferred brand: NutriBiotic) — 1/4 tsp.

HOW TO DO IT:
Scoop the Seasoap out of jar and place it into a mixing bowl. Add the other ingredients one at a time in order, mixing by hand to avoid excessive foaming.

HOW TO USE IT:
This is an excellent everyday shampoo for babies and children. We also recommend this formula for adults with skin and scalp sensitivities. Note: Do

not get shampoo into baby's eyes, as even natural soaps can cause irritation. (This is not a vegan formula.) IMPORTANT: Keep refrigerated when not in use.

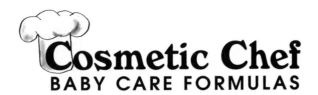

Cosmetic Chef
BABY CARE FORMULAS

FORMULA #30
Natural Baby's Evening Primrose Lotion

A **baby's skin is extremely sensitive.** Many infants suffer from eczema and a number of skin irritations, including the inevitable bouts of diaper rash, but these problems are easily corrected. This soothing lotion is very similar to my Evening Primrose Hand and Body Lotion for problem skin (Formula #16), but is much milder, especially formulated to help heal and pamper a baby's ultra-delicate skin.

INGREDIENTS:

Tofu Essential Fatty Acid Cream Base (Formula #1) — 1 cup
Aloe Vera Gel (preferred brand: Aubrey Organics®, or fresh gel from aloe
   plant — just remove fillet from leaf and liquefy in blender) — 1/2 cup
Evening Primrose Oil (preferred brand: Aubrey Organics®) — 2 tsp.
White Camellia Oil (preferred brand: Aubrey Organics®) — 2 tsp.
Flaxseed Oil (preferred brands: Barleans, Arrowhead Mills) — 2 tsp.
Jojoba Oil (preferred brand: Aubrey Organics®) — 2 tsp.
Aubrey Organics® Angelica Eau de Cologne (optional) — 4 drops

HOW TO DO IT:

Make the Tofu Essential Fatty Acid Cream Base and place it in a bowl. Add the other ingredients in the order shown, one at a time. Using a hand mixer or blender, blend together until you get a smooth cream. Finish with 4 drops of Angelica Eau de Cologne (the fragrance is optional, but very pleasant).

HOW TO USE IT:

This baby lotion is far superior than any you can buy in drug stores or department stores because it contains no synthetics that can be absorbed into baby's skin and cause allergic reactions and other more serious health problems. It is an excellent treatment for rashes, eczema and other skin disorders. Note: Remember never to use bath powder, which can be inhaled into baby's lungs, or mineral oil, which is harsh and drying to the skin. IMPORTANT: Keep refrigerated when not in use.

VI

Things To Look For,
Things To Avoid in
Your Cosmetic Products

At some point we have all been seduced by a slick ad campaign touting some amazing product that will change our lives. Imagine sitting at your dressing table at night, unscrewing the jar and dipping your fingers deep into that miracle potion that will turn back the clock on your skin, clear up all forms of acne and blemishes, erase any lines and imperfections and restore your complexion's youthful elasticity, all before breakfast the next morning! Admit it. The only real miracle about this product is the fact that they've persuaded you to buy it at all.

Now consider this reality check: Imagine the 50,000 gallon vats in which the product was mixed, the petrochemical factory where the raw materials were coaxed out of the coal tar or mineral oil, the long assembly line where the elaborately printed bottles (which cost many times more than the ingredients that went into them) were filled, capped and boxed. Production of this kind was unheard of 100 years ago. But can you honestly say that the mass manufacture of cosmetics has caused an outbreak of ageless beauty? Your hair and skin are a living testimony to the successes and failures of mass-produced cosmetics. Most of us don't like what we see.

These days when you read the label on a cosmetic product, you practically need a Ph.D. in chemistry to identify most of the ingredients. But it doesn't take a rocket scientist to recognize that these multi-syllabic tongue twisters aren't in the mix to improve your quality of life. Preservatives such as methyl and propyl paraben aren't there to protect you—they are added to save cosmetic manufacturers money and keep their formulas intact on warehouse shelves for periods of up to three years or more!

Preservatives are just one class of chemicals needed for effective mass manufacturing of cosmetic products. Emulsifiers, foam-builders, sequestering agents (which help cosmetics hold their color) and synthetic colors and fragrances are other classes, each with its own particular set of demands mass production imposes. None of them have anything to do with improving the health of your hair and skin. You're putting all this chemical technology on your body, but what is it really doing for you? Are there safer ingredients that can work just as well without exposing you to so many toxic chemicals? You already know the answer to that question, or you wouldn't be reading this book in the first place.

Megan Shields, M.D., family specialist and internationally recognized expert in detoxification therapies and low-toxin living (whose work appears in such scientific journals as *Ambio*, published by the Royal Swedish Academy of Sciences), shares her views on the difference between natural and synthetic ingredients. She wrote to us:

"As a family health physician who also specializes in helping patients overcome both environmental and occupational chemical exposures, I'm very concerned about the types of consumer products that people bring into their homes. One area of particular concern is the cosmetics and personal care products that my patients pick up from the local drug and department stores. I mean, here they've come into my office and taken extra special steps to clean up their lifestyle, their diet, to start exercising and minimizing their use of unsafe prescription medications—and then they go out and purchase a cosmetic product with formaldehyde-releasing preservatives, eye irritants, allergens and other toxins! It just doesn't make sense to be applying this stuff to your skin and reintroducing it into your system when you've taken so much care to get it out of your body. That's why I stress to my patients the health virtues of natural cosmetics, whether made at home or purchased from their local health food store. I'd much rather see my patients applying green tea and milk thistle to their skin than quaternium-15 or some other toxic compound!"

The quaternium-15 Dr. Shields singles out above is a quaternary ammonium salt. When you use a hair conditioner or cream rinse that contains it, you are putting on your hair a chemical used in the paper and fabric industries as a softener and antistatic agent. It can also be used as a water repellent, fungicide, emulsifier and corrosion inhibitor. The quaternary ammonium compounds are toxic and do not belong on your hair and skin.

David Steinman, author of *Diet for a Poisoned Planet* (Ballantine, 1992), co-author of *The Safe Shopper's Bible* (Macmillan, 1995), and publisher of the newsletter *The Doctors' Prescription for Healthy Living* wrote the following to us concerning the use of chemicals in cosmetics:

"The ultimate criteria for a consumer product is that it not only work, but that it be proven safe for general use. Unfortunately, most drug store and high-end brands of shampoo and skin products do not meet this criteria. The recent scientific findings from the federal National Toxicology Program on the carcinogenicity of free diethanolamine (DEA) in cosmetic products raises special concerns. Take shampoos, which so frequently use this chemical toxin. The combination of warm water and cleanser makes the skin even more permeable and allows for even greater absorption of toxins. What's more, if diethanolamine mixes with nitrites (also found in some shampoo and skin lotion products, although not disclosed on labels), the combination can be even more deadly by causing formation of a second set of proven carcinogens called nitrosamines. As diethanolamine and triethanolamine (TEA, which contains free diethanolamine) are so frequently used in commercial drug store and high-end brands of shampoos and skin lotions, I urge my patients to seek a safe, natural approach to health and beauty.

"Natural cosmetics, whether homemade or purchased from select national leaders in the natural product industry, avoid these kinds of toxic pitfalls. Instead, they rely on herbal ingredients, combined with nutrients and other safe, natural substances that have a proven record of efficacy and safety. What's more, my own experience and that of my family indicates that natural is better when it comes to looking and feeling your best."

In the best of all possible worlds you would never expect that by using a shampoo, you could actually be introducing cancer-causing nitrosamines into your body. But as David Steinman points out here and in many of his books, DEA is a toxic chemical that should definitely be avoided.

L. Stephen Coles, M.D., Ph.D., specialist in obstetrics and gynecology, and a well-known longevity expert who serves on the editorial board of *The Journal of Anti-Aging Medicine,* also wrote to us on the topic of chemical additives in cosmetics:

"What most people don't realize is that the skin is like a human sink which absorbs the toxins in commercial cosmetic and personal care products. I'm so concerned about this that I tell all my patients to always seek safe and healthy natural cosmetics. Sometimes I even show them myself how they can make a great conditioner for their hair simply by using the milk protein found in yogurt, or how they can create highlights in their hair with the use of certain safe herbal preparations, or how ginseng works as a scalp stimulant, and biotin actually helps to thicken the hair. There are all sorts of techniques and tricks that consumers can learn to make their own great cosmetics. For kids, I always recommend the natural route, since their skin is even more susceptible to the allergens and irritants in commercial cosmetics and will respond even more favorably to natural cosmetics and personal care products."

Gary Wilkholm, M.D., family practice specialist and medical advisory board member of *The Doctors' Prescription for Healthy Living,* had this to say:

"As the author of a book that uncovered the dirty secrets of the cosmetic industry, I know firsthand that commercial cosmetic products may be loaded with chemical toxins that increase your risk for allergies, irritation, and even cancer. By learning the secrets of making your own natural cosmetics and personal care products, you'll not only save money and have fun making them, you'll be going a long way toward detoxifying your skin from the many unsafe chemicals in cosmetic products. Ginseng, biotin, mucopolysaccharides, coltsfoot, horsetail, yucca, quillaya bark, rosemary—these are the ingredients of safe and healthy beauty."

Another expert in the field, Dr. C. Leigh Broadhurst, Ph.D., visiting scientist at USDA Beltsville Human Nutrition Research Center and Environmental Chemistry Laboratory in Maryland, wrote to us at great length on this subject. Dr. Broadhurst is President of 22nd Century Nutrition, Inc., as well as Nutrition and Scientific Consulting Vice-President for Herbal Vineyard, Inc. This is what she had to say about natural cosmetics versus synthetic:

"I have used Aubrey Organics® skin and hair care products for myself and my family for about 10 years. I use them because they are a wonderful mix of art and science, and that mix provides beautiful results with a very minimal risk of skin/scalp allergies and irritations. I remember using a shampoo in high school that was popular and that all my friends used. After a few uses, I broke out in a horrible, pimply, red rash on my neck, back and scalp. Years later one of Aubrey's books educated me on the fact that my shampoo had contained formaldehyde, and I was one of thousands suffering from similar reactions.

"On the scientific front I'm a chemist, and one of my major areas of research is in polyunsaturated fatty acids, sometimes called essential fatty acids, or EFA's. EFA's are essential nutritional fats, meaning that they can't be made by the body and must be consumed in the diet. EFA's are highly concentrated in the skin, and a deficiency of them causes dry, scaly, itchy skin, dry, dull hair, brittle nails and excessive thirst due to the fact that the skin cannot prevent the body's water from evaporating as it should.

"It's not well-known, but EFA's can be directly absorbed by the skin, especially in infants. It's not a good idea to simply slather EFA oils on your skin and not bother to take them internally, but neither is it a good idea to take a spoonful of flaxseed oil per day and hope for the best, relying on petroleum-based skin lotions to correct your dry skin.

"From a chemical standpoint, it makes no sense to use petroleum-based hydrocarbon oils and waxes as skin moisturizers. Our skin oils are not anywhere near this type of fat composition. The reason why petroleum jelly feels "greasy" is because it does not dissolve into our skin's natural oils—it just sits on top of the skin. This may keep water from evaporating in the short term, but it does nothing to actually improve and repair the condition of the skin—this takes EFA's. A truly beneficial moisturizer (1) contains natural vegetable oils (2) contains EFA's (3) blends quickly and easily into the skin, and is never greasy (4) causes no short term or long term irritations (5) actually improves the condition of the skin so that less moisturizer is needed per day, not more. In point 5, only honest companies like Aubrey Organics® would have you use less of a product, not more!

"The art comes in along with the science in Aubrey's use of botanicals. Everyone must think of skin lotions, hair conditioners, etc., *exactly* the same way they think of foods. The components in these cosmetic products can and do get absorbed into the skin/hair, and you can "feed" your skin and hair a junk food diet, or you can feed it a natural, organic, whole "food" diet. Genus *Homo* is 2.5 million years old, and fully modern *Homo sapiens* (us humans!) have been around since between 100,000 and 300,000 years ago. This is a *very* long time compared to the 50 or 100 years that refined, processed and "junk" foods have been around, and since synthetic moisturizers, detergents, humectants, emulsifiers, perfumes, colors and antimicrobials have been around. Our bodies haven't had anywhere near enough time to get used to eating artificial colors and flavors, cereal grains, sugar and hydrogenated fats. Neither have they had enough time to get used to synthetic cosmetic chemicals and fats. On the other hand, natural botanical products have been used by humans since day one, and they absolutely are both more effective and less allergenic. I have two small children now, and the first baths I gave them as newborns were with Aubrey's Natural Baby Bath Soap, because I knew I could trust it on their sensitive skin.

"Botanical ingredients are more expensive, but result in a more effective and safer product. They also result in a more pleasant, wholesome product. There's always some art and folklore involved in choosing combinations of herbs that not only do the job, but look and smell attractive, and have synergy when blended. This only comes with trial and error, experience, and a real love and commitment to the design of herbal products. I don't see another major company in the natural products industry who goes as far in this direction as Aubrey Organics®."

It was kind of Dr. Broadhurst to recommend our products, but more important is her story concerning formaldehyde in the shampoo she used. A cosmetic can have formaldehyde in it, but you won't see it on the label. Formaldehyde can be formed by a preservative such as Germall II (Diazolidinyl urea) and Germall 115 (Imidazolidinyl urea). You'll often see these names on the labels of a cosmetic product, but you might not know that at a temperature of $10°$ C, this chemical releases formaldehyde into the product. These chemicals are toxic and often result in serious rashes on the skin much like the ones Dr. Broadhurst experienced with the mass-produced shampoo she mentioned earlier.

Marcus Laux, N.D., professor and staff physician at the College of Naturopathic Medicine in Portland, OR, wrote the following on why natural cosmetics are better for you:

"I've been in practice since 1985 and, without exception, natural hair and skin care products are what I recommend for my patients, my friends, my family and myself. There is no doubt in my mind that whatever touches your skin ends up in your body. It can help you or hurt you. I have found that natural hair and skin care products—when they are truly natural—feel better on the skin, and cause fewer problems such as rashes or other allergic responses.

"In private practice, many patients come in with problems, skin rashes, allergies and skin conditions that look like atopic dermatitis. Often after going through their history, I make a few changes in their diet, change their choice of personal care products, and together we watch a lot of these problems go away.

"Using natural hair and skin care products means that we're not just *not* polluting the environment, but we're also using something that is great for us. Natural products are also so much more luxurious. The real smells of the plant extracts and the essential oils, the feel of the products that are less refined but no less elegant, are unforgettable treats. My baby has only known natural products. My wife and I have used natural products for decades. We consciously feel so much better and happier, in our right stance with the planet, with the universe."

What to Look for, What to Avoid

What follows is some good, solid advice on which ingredients to look for and which to stay away from when shopping for your cosmetic products. We can't list all the harmful chemicals used by the cosmetic industry, but we've singled out some of the worst offenders and provided safe, natural alternatives to help you make wiser and more health-friendly choices in the future.

AVOID:

Diethanolamine—More commonly known as DEA, this synthetic chemical turns up in most commercial shampoos as a wetting agent. You often see it combined with coconut oil soap, and listed as Cocamide DEA. Like triethanolamine (TEA), it may be contaminated with nitrosamines, known to be potent carcinogens. These cancer-causing compounds are formed when nitrates are combined with amines (organic nitrogen compounds), and are absorbed by the skin in amounts far greater than when eating nitrate-preserved foods. In his book *Consumer's Guide to Cosmetics* (Anchor Doubleday, 1980), Tom Conry points out that, "Although not all TEA- or DEA-containing cosmetics are nitrosamine-contaminated, the consumer has no way of determining which products are safe... The most prudent course would be to avoid DEA and TEA." In the 1980s, the FDA tested commercial products containing DEA and TEA and found that 37% of the products tested contained carcinogenic nitrosamine impurities.

LOOK FOR:

Vegetable Glycerine—Used in cosmetic formulations for thousands of years, vegetable glycerine makes an excellent wetting agent. It does the job naturally and effectively, without any toxic side effects. Sometimes, but not always, shampoos and soaps without DEA and TEA will be slightly thinner and have a lighter sudsing action that those containing these chemicals. They will clean your hair as well or better than a chemicalized, high suds product. Remember, a little less suds is a better alternative than allowing potential carcinogens to be absorbed into your body through your skin and scalp.

AVOID:

Mineral Oil—Here's a chemical you see on almost every moisturizer, usually as one of the top three ingredients. This petroleum derivative is harsh on the skin and has been known to cause severe allergic reactions, but it's a cheap alternative to natural oils, and cosmetic manufacturers can't pass up a bargain! When you first put it on it leaves a greasy feel, but its molecules are so large, the oil stays on top of your skin and over time tends to dry it out and cause pores to become clogged. Mineral oil is actually bottled and sold as a baby oil, but take our word for it—the last thing you'll want to do is put it on your baby. The only place this petrochemical belongs is in the crankcase of your car engine, not on your skin.

LOOK FOR:

Jojoba Oil—This fabulous moisturizer is the natural extract from the jojoba plant, commonly found in Arizona and Mexico. The rich, waxy oil that collects in the jojoba beans actually helps this hardy desert plant attract and retain moisture during the long drought, allowing it to withstand summer temperatures of up to 115°! It works similarly on your hair and skin by helping to seal moisture in.

Rosa Mosqueta® Rose Hip Seed Oil—The oil extract from the rose hip seeds of this rare South American rose is extremely high in essential fatty acids, necessary for skin cell regeneration, as well as vitamin C, and its healing and moisturizing properties are nothing short of miraculous. Clinical tests have shown that when applied to damaged skin, it speeds up the healing process and helps fade or prevent scarring. Ideal for dry or mature skin, it diminishes the appearance of fine lines and wrinkles and improves texture. It also makes an excellent hot oil treatment for dry, brittle hair and split ends.

AVOID:

Propylene Glycol—This is the synthetic form of glycerine, derived from propylene alcohol and highly irritating to the skin and scalp. In cosmetic formulas it acts as an emulsifier (keeping the oil and water phases of a cosmetic from separating) and a humectant. It is another petrochemical—not exactly a blessing to our environment— and a major cause of allergic reactions, clogged pores and blemishes.

LOOK FOR:

Vegetable Glycerine — Natural glycerine is great for attracting moisture to your skin, and is easily absorbed, acting as a carrying agent for herbs and other nutrients. We recommend vegetable glycerine in many of the formulas in this book, as both a moisturizer and an emulsifier.

AVOID:

Sodium Lauryl Sulfate/Sodium Laureth Sulfate (SLS)—Just as mineral oil is found in most moisturizers, creams and lotions, these two synthetic chemicals are included in nearly all mass-produced shampoos, and even in many brands of toothpaste! They are synthetic detergents and foam builders, quaintly known in the industry as "syndets." Although you'll find them in many so-called "natural" cosmetics with the explanation "from coconut oil," they are not natural—they're synthetically produced through what is known as the Ziegler process, and rarely come from coconuts. To make matters worse, SLS is often used in combination with triethanolamine (TEA) which, as we discussed earlier, can be contaminated with cancer-causing nitrosamines. Plus SLS is bad for the environment, polluting our water supply when it goes down the drain.

LOOK FOR:

Natural Soaps (Coconut Oil [Cocamide without DEA], Olive Oil Castile, Quillaya or Yucca Root Soaps)—In order to avoid the petrochemicals found in most shampoos, simply look for formulas made with any of these natural soaps. These are the original liquid soaps and the first shampoos, made from natural substances through a saponification reaction with salt. They may have a slightly lower sudsing action than their synthetic equivalents, but are much gentler on your hair and skin and don't pollute the environment or your body with toxic chemicals. We use them as a base in our recipes for natural shampoos, soaps and cleansers.

AVOID:

Methyl and Propyl Paraben—These are commonly used cosmetic preservatives, also known as p-hydroxybenzoate (or PHB) esters. Like hexachlorophene (the antibacterial we discussed earlier that caused brain damage in babies), they are designed to kill bacteria and extend the shelf life of products for several years. They are very toxic, a leading cause of contact dermatitis, and are incompatible with many types of shampoo bases, as well as protein (such as collagen). Parabens are also not particularly effective against microorganisms and fungi.

Imidazolidinyl Urea—This synthetic preservative is most frequently used in shampoos, but can also be found in other cosmetics. Its purpose in a cleanser is to "bind" with metallic ions so they will not interfere with the cleansing action of the shampoo or soap. The most serious side effect is that it releases formaldehyde into the product (as we discussed earlier in this chapter). Here's a list of other chemicals with the same formaldehyde-releasing properties: 2-bromo-2-nitropropane-1,3-diol; diazolidinyl urea; DMDM hydantoin; Quaternium-15.

LOOK FOR:

Grapefruit Seed Extract (Citrus Seed Extract) and Vitamins A, C and E—First used as a cosmetic preservative in the 1970s, grapefruit seed extract is widely effective against fungi, bacteria and other microorganisms in both water- and oil-based products. When combined with antioxidant vitamins A, C and E, grapefruit seed extract keeps both water- and oil-based cosmetics stable for a year or more. It is a highly effective and widely tolerated natural preservative.

AVOID:

Lanolin—Lanolin is the fatty secretion from sheep's wool. While it has been known to cause allergic reactions in some people, a more serious problem with this animal byproduct is that it can be contaminated with DDT, dieldrin, lindane and other neurotoxic and carcinogenic pesticides. According to David Steinman and Samuel Epstein, M.D., *(The Safe Shopper's Bible)*, in 1988 as many as 16 pesticides were identified in lanolin. (The neurotoxic organophosphate pesticide diazinon was found in 21 out of 25 samples of lanolin!) The National Academy of Sciences has expressed concern that, due to the fact that lanolin is a powerful absorbing agent, topical application could cause these highly toxic pesticides to be easily absorbed into the bloodstream.

LOOK FOR:

Essential Oils—Essential oils are superb emollients with therapeutic effects on both the hair and scalp. Jojoba oil in particular is an ideal substitute. More a "liquid wax" than an oil, it has a similar consistency to lanolin, and adds shine and manageability to the hair (the main reasons lanolin is used in hair care products). White camellia and Rosa Mosqueta® oils, discussed earlier, are also excellent choices.

AVOID:

Talc—Absurdly enough, talc is still used as a powder for babies, although it is a known carcinogen when breathed into the lungs. Another startling fact is that talc, commonly used around a baby's genital area, has been linked to ovarian cancer. Don't use it at all.

LOOK FOR:

Corn Starch or Rice Starch Powder—There are any number of powders that can replace talc. They are just as effective and are far safer. (For a superb baby lotion with evening primrose oil to help fight and prevent diaper rash, see Formula #30 in Part V.)

AVOID:

Silica— Silica is used in creams and lotions to thicken the product and stabilize emulsions, and in powdered cosmetics to enhance flow (in some cosmetic powders you may be getting both talc and silica at the same time). Like talc, silica can cause fibrosis of the lung and other respiratory disorders, and should be avoided. It can also contain small amounts of crystallized quartz, a known carcinogen. You don't need silica in your cosmetics—say no to any product that contains it.

LOOK FOR:

Psyllium Husks Powder and Lecithin—Both psyllium husks powder and lecithin are safe, natural thickeners and emulsifiers.

AVOID:

Sodium PCA (NaPCA)—This chemical is a sodium salt of pyroglutamic acid, often used in skin conditioners and moisturizers. The marketing angle is that it is very similar to substances in our skin and acts as a natural moisturizing factor. It does not. It can cause strong allergic reactions and can severely dry out your skin by absorbing moisture from it.

LOOK FOR:

Pantothenic Acid (Panthenol)—This B vitamin is an excellent nutrient and skin softener that attracts moisture to the skin and is safe to use in any cosmetic formula. It is a great humectant in both hair and skin care products. Vegetable glycerine is another safer and better moisturizer.

AVOID:

Synthetic Hair Dyes—Regular use of synthetic hair colors is strongly associated with a significant risk of cancer (this is particularly true of dark hair dyes). Avoid dye products containing phenylenediamine. Bleaching the hair is safer, though solutions may be harsh and can leave hair dry and damaged.

LOOK FOR:

Henna—Vegetable-based hair dyes, such as henna, are much safer and gentler on your hair. There is no cancer risk associated with henna-based hair products. Many different shades are available; plus, henna has an excellent conditioning effect, and is particularly beneficial for limp, lackluster hair and oily scalp.

AVOID:

Synthetic Fragrances—May be a blend of up to 600 different chemicals, few of which have been tested for human toxicity. A primary cause of irritation, photosensitivity and allergic reactions. There is also a cancer risk, since very little is known of fragrance constituents.

LOOK FOR:

Natural Fragrances—There's no guarantee you won't have an allergic reaction to a natural fragrance, but the primary culprits are well known and are not frequently used any more. Natural fragrances are mostly essential oils from herbs and flowers. Not only do they add to the experience of using a cosmetic product, but essential oils have a therapeutic effect on the hair and skin, and are used in aromatherapy treatments for their soothing and centering properties on both the body and the mind.

AVOID:

PVP-VA/Copolymers—Widely used in hairsprays and styling gels, these are actually plastics, which coat the hair and make it look dull and lifeless. But more importantly, they can be considered toxic, particularly when minute particles are inhaled into the lungs, where they may cause all sorts of respiratory problems.

LOOK FOR:

Herbal Gums—Acacia and tragacanth gums have been used in hair care products for many centuries. Dissolved, they can be used as hairsprays and styling gels, or added to "body building" shampoos for thin, limp hair. They are particularly effective when combined with panthenol (vitamin B-5), a natural hair thickener and humectant that adds body and fullness without leaving the hair gummy and hard to the touch. A recent addition to the natural "film forming agents" is Larex®, a trade name for Larch gum, which is harvested from the unused portions of the Larch tree. In 1993 Michael Finney, president of Larex, Inc., introduced this unique natural polymer, which easily replaces synthetic copolymers and is ideal for holding a hair style naturally.

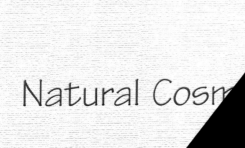

Natural Cosm

VII

The Top Ten
(plus one)
...letic Companies

Here we go—out on a limb. Since we've been involved in manufacturing and researching cosmetic products for a long time, we always get the "dirt." Consumers write us all the time to tell us which cosmetics they've found to cause the most problems, as well as which products do the best job on their hair and skin. Over the years we've gotten a "feel" for the field with these thousands of letters of praise and blame (and they all name brand names). While it's useless to point fingers, there are ways you can protect yourself from unethical companies and shoddy manufacturing practices.

What You Need to Know About Cosmetic Manufacturers

There was a time in America when we bought from a company not only because we believed in the quality of its products and ingredients, but also because that company stood for something that was important to us. Sadly, this trusting relationship between company and consumer has largely disappeared. Today consumers are much more skeptical, and with good reason. When choosing your cosmetics, there are some important questions you should ask yourself, not only about the products, but about the companies that make them.

You can tell a great deal about a company's integrity just by reading the ingredients labels on their products. How many tongue-twisting, chemical-sounding names do you see? Is the product description copy on the label full of the latest "buzz words?" Are they jumping on the "what's hot" bandwagon and pushing the latest fad ingredients? (Alpha-hydroxy and super-vitamin C are big ones right now.) How do their prices compare with the types of ingredients being offered?

Reading the label of the product you are considering buying is important, but that won't tell you the whole story. Be sure to also look at the labels of several other cosmetics made by that same company to see just how far their commitment to quality ingredients really goes.

How Green are They Really?

We've talked at great length about the many synthetic chemicals that have been created over the past 60 years, and how they impact not only our bodies but the world we live in. An ethical cosmetic manufacturer will also care about the environment and do his/her part to address these concerns in their manufacturing practices as well as in their choice of ingredients.

One example of this is packaging. Obviously, from an environmental standpoint, glass bottles are superior to plastic, but in terms of shipping costs (glass is heavier and much more expensive to ship) and safety (think of keeping a glass shampoo bottle in your shower), it is not always practical. However, many socially responsible companies use HDPE plastic bottles, which are not only more cost-effective, but fully recyclable.

One environmental buzz word that is frequently overused in the industry is "biodegradable." This simply means the product can be broken down and assimilated by nature. Still, many so-called biodegradable cosmetic or household cleaning products contain synthetic detergents, preservatives and other harmful ingredients, so as they break down, they put these potentially toxic chemicals into the earth. This is hardly a responsible way to make products, and to try and promote this as something good for the environment only adds insult to injury.

Choosing Your Products

When choosing your cosmetics, some people recommend you look for products with as few ingredients as possible. While this is a good rule of thumb, some products contain long lists of ingredients—particularly herbals—that are very beneficial for your hair and skin.

Once you've purchased the product, doing your own personal patch test is important, because you may be allergic to some natural ingredient that sounds harmless enough. If you know you have a food allergy to a particular ingredient—milk, for example—then chances are you will be allergic to milk or a milk byproduct used as an ingredient in a cosmetic. When trying out a new product, first take a small amount of the contents and rub it on the inside of your arm. Put a bandage over it for 24 hours, then examine the area. Is there any redness or a rash? If there is no adverse reaction, then it's very likely you can use the product with no problems.

Hypoallergenic is, for the most part, a bogus term. One of the top cosmetic companies that uses this word to promote its products includes many synthetic ingredients in its formulas that are known sensitizers and very harsh for the skin (as well as harmful to the environment). Products labeled as "hypoallergenic" are not necessarily safe to use, and are often full of synthetic chemicals known to cause allergic reactions and other health problems.

Buy from Someone You Trust

The good news is that there are some very good companies making excellent natural cosmetics. Because we know you can't always make your own cosmetic products at home, we want to tell you about a few of them. Although the method of manufacture and the purity of ingredients were our primary litmus test, we also took other things into account when selecting these companies. For instance, we are aware that Jill Nadine Clements, of Nadine's Creams, gives work to physically challenged people in the packaging plant of her cosmetic company. And we remember Paul Penders was the first cosmetic manufacturer to place ads touting that his natural products are "cruelty-free." We also recommend these companies because the people who run them have values we think are commendable.

What follows is a list of some highly respected manufacturers making quality, natural cosmetics in a responsible way. This list is not exactly comprehensive; it's limited to those companies we are familiar with. More than likely, somewhere out there exists a cosmetic manufacturer making a fabulous, all-natural face cream that's great for your skin, and we simply don't know about it. (If this is the case, please write and let us know.) The companies mentioned here are good, ethical cosmetic manufacturers we feel you can trust. These are simply our recommendations, based on what we know of their track record and what we have observed through the years. As with all recommendations, remember ours are rather subjective, given with the best of intentions, and far from foolproof, so use your own judgement.

The Top Ten (Plus One) Cosmetic Manufacturers We Recommend
(Listed Alphabetically)

Alexandra Avery Purely Natural Body Care
4717 S. E. Belmont St.
Portland, OR 97215
TEL: (800) 669-1863 — FAX: (503) 236-5926
Website: www.gaines.com

The lovely array of products from this small, Oregon-based company came wrapped in lavender paper, a colorful way to introduce you to this fragrant line. The company's founder—yes, there is an Alexandra Avery—was born in Hawaii. As a child, her company bio tells us, she enjoyed "hosting flower feasts in tree forts along the beach." Sounds idyllic, doesn't it? But her childhood pastime became her adult livelihood with the creation of her bodycare company in 1976. Today, her 100% natural range of products has strong roots in aromatherapy, with complex yet delicate blends such as Jungle Blossom Body Oil and Underactive Skin Elixir. These feature essential oils in a mixture of safflower, sesame and sweet almond oils. Another great product is a delightful Aromatherapy Toner with witch hazel, aloe vera, vegetable glycerine, rosewater, orange oil, St. John's wort, calendula and other herbals. The line also includes creams, dry masks, scented body powders, soaps and cleansers.

The company has received several awards for its purity and efficacy. Further, it was one of six small businesses to be named in the "honor roll" of the Council on Economic Priorities book, *Shopping for a Better World.* Alexandra's book *Aromatherapy and You: A Guide to Natural Skin Care*, is an aromatic adventure of essential facts about natural skin care.

Aubrey Organics®, Inc.
4419 N. Manhattan Ave.
Tampa, FL 33614
TEL: (800) 282-7394
TEL: (813) 877-4186 — FAX: (813) 876-8166
Website: www.aubrey-organics.com

Aubrey Organics® was started in New York City in 1967 by Aubrey Hampton with a product called Relax-R-Bath. More than 30 years later, Aubrey has created a wide variety of hair and skin care products handcrafted in his Tampa, Florida plant and sold all over the world. Aubrey first learned about natural cosmetics from his mother, a second generation French woman who settled in southern Indiana and made her own hair and skin care products from herbs she grew herself (see How This Book Came About in the Preface). Aubrey helped her make all kinds of cosmetic products at home, and later put this ability to work, formulating and manufacturing more than 200 hair, skin and bodycare products. Aubrey Organics® is the only certified organic cosmetic manufacturer in the United States (as of this writing). This extensive line is available in health food stores around the United States and Canada, as well as on their web site and through direct mail.

Aubrey Organics® is unique in its method of manufacture: products are made in small batches of 50 gallons or less, and are never warehoused. Instead they are shipped directly to health food stores and consumers without a middleman, thereby guaranteeing customers the freshest products at the best possible prices.

In the 1970s Aubrey pioneered the use of natural preservatives with his citrus seed extract and vitamins A, C and E blend, as well as the use of many herbals in cosmetics, including Rosa Mosqueta® rose hip seed oil, blue camomile oil, white camellia oil, shea butter, evening primrose oil and calaguala fern extract. Some of Aubrey's top-selling products are GPB (Glycogen Protein Balancer) Hair Conditioner and Nutrient, a hair conditioner made with milk protein, rosemary and sage extracts, balsam tolu and sulfur-containing amino acids; Blue Camomile Shampoo, a mild hair cleanser formulated with rare blue camomile oil from Morocco; Natural & Herbal Facial Cleanser, with menthol, camphor and eucalyptus extracts; and Rosa Mosqueta® Rose Hip Moisturizing Cream, a rich skin-nourisher and revitalizer.

Autumn Harp, Inc.
61 Pine St.
Bristol. VT 05443,
TEL: (802) 453-4807 — FAX: (802) 453-4203

Autumn Harp is known for its petroleum-free products, which means you won't find all those terrible petrochemicals in their cosmetics, and that's a good thing. Kevin Harper, the man who founded Autumn Harp in 1976, is committed to all-natural products that are good for the body and safe for the environment. Manufactured in an 11,000 square foot state-of-the-art plant in rural Vermont, Autumn Harp makes a wide variety of lip balms and salves under their famous Un-Petroleum brand name. It all started with Un-Petroleum Jelly, a unique blend of castor oil, coconut oil, beeswax, silica and vitamin E, which blows its synthetic, petroleum-based counterparts out of the water. It moisturizes, soothes and protects, all with plant-based ingredients. Today, Kevin makes Un-Petroleum Lip Balm, Medicated Lip Spice and Sunscreen Lip Balm, as well as a line of lip products for children. Ingredients used, besides those mentioned above, include candellia wax, Brazil nut oil, jojoba oil, aloe vera, carnauba wax, meadow foam seed oil and a variety of natural flavors. Kevin also makes products for the Body Shop and has been responsible for some of its best-selling items.

Autumn Harp is a company that looks beyond trendy "green marketing" and towards changing the way business works in the world. As company president Paul Ralson states, "We want customers who not only value our products for the quality we put into them, but who know us and support our efforts to provide an alternative to the cosmetic industry's dependency on synthetic and petroleum products."

Dr. Bronner's All One God's Faith, Inc.
P. O. Box 28
Escondido, CA 92033
TEL: (760) 743-2211 — FAX: (760) 745-6675
Website: www.drbronner.com

Throughout this book we have cautioned the reader to read cosmetic labels; many of them list words so long you can barely pronounce them, and the ingredients look like a mad chemist's dream. Not so with Dr. Bronner's. This most unique man is a purist who learned the soap business from his parents in Germany, and his wonderful products are about as natural as they come. If you are concerned about "overpackaging" and "glitz," you won't get it from this company. "He's got a label like the Holy Bible," comments one person on picking up Dr. Bronner's Castile Peppermint Soap for the first time. His labels do have inspirational religious quotes—there are plenty of them, and you'll have to get out your magnifying glass to read them all. His son, James Bronner, carries on in the same ethical vein as his father, a "chip off the old block."

Dr. Bronner's liquid soaps are among the best you can buy. They contains none of the synthetic detergents, foam-builders and synthetic preservatives (no DEA or TEA!) found in most formulations. His castile soap comes in the original peppermint as well as almond, lavender, eucalyptus and a fragrant blend they call "baby soap."

Dr. Hauschka Cosmetics U.S.A., Inc.
59C North St.
Hatfield, MA 01038
TEL: (413) 247-9907 — FAX: (413) 247-0608

Dr. Hauschka Cosmetics are made by WALA, a cruelty-free cosmetic manufacturer that has been popular in Germany and throughout Europe for many years. WALA offers a complete line of holistic preparations formulated with organic and biodynamically grown plants that encourage the healthy functioning of the skin. It is known in particular for its bath elixirs, which use only the finest essential oil blends.

WALA has been cultivating biodynamic gardens for over 40 years and also supports biodynamic initiatives throughout the world. Biodynamic methods of agriculture take into account the ecology of the earth as a whole, as well as its relationship to the universe. The goal of biodynamic farming is to heal the earth for generations to come. Biodynamically grown plants carry vital nutrients that encourage the skin to balance itself and become active. WALA uses environmentally sound, rhythmical processing to strengthen and preserve the living essence of its plant-based ingredients. This ensures that no aspect of nature is damaged in the process, including plants, animals or people.

Susan West Kurz points out that their formulas meet all skin needs, addressing specific skin conditions rather than skin types due to the fact that the skin has the ability to change, to become more balanced and harmonious.

"Through biodynamic agriculture, rhythmic processing and preparations that support the healthy functioning of the skin, we treat the skin as the royal robe of humankind. It is a balanced, holistic approach to skin care," Ms. Kurz continues. "It is what happens when you allow science and spirit to work together."

We've found that there are many excellent natural products in the Dr. Hauschka Cosmetics line, and their dedication to natural formulas makes most selections among the very best for your skin. Three skin care products (for three skin care steps) particularly appealed to us: Dr. Hauschka Cleansing Cream is formulated with the nuts and shells of sweet almonds to provide a gentle exfoliation especially effective on sensitive skin; Dr. Hauschka Face Lotion gives the skin a fresh feeling and has a "toning" effect; Dr. Hauschka Skin Conditioner works well on all skin types and leaves the complexion soft and smooth, and is particularly recommended for complexions that show signs of premature aging. Dr. Hauschka's chemical-free lipsticks are also excellent, and their Cream Foundations (which come in dark, bronze and medium colors) contain none of the harsh synthetics used in most makeups that can cause contact dermatitis or acne.

Geremy Rose
PO Box 1947
Brattleboro, VT 05301
TEL: (802) 257-0018 — FAX: (802) 257-0652
Website: www.newchapterinc.com

Paul Schulick started this natural cosmetic company in 1989 and named it after his two children. He is an herbalist, so he knows quite a bit about which herbs are the most beneficial for hair and skin. His products are natural and original, and you can be assured you're not just getting the latest "buzz word" ingredients in his formulas, which are worth every dollar you spend. Paul takes his inspiration from the ancient use of botanicals in skin care, an approach he calls "fresh skin care," based on the idea that the power of herbs and botanical foods rests in their potency—their freshness. Products are naturally preserved with essential oils and herbal extracts and shipped UPS two-day directly to stores outside the Northeast, so you can be assured of their freshness.

Although small, this product line is complete, and one of the best-organized we've seen. Each product is labeled as either (1) cleanser or mask, (2) toner, (3) moisturizer or (4) treatment. Products are then subdivided into what's appropriate for individual skin types, including normal, oily, sensitive, dry, mature and blemish-prone skin. This system allows the customer to choose quickly and easily which product is best for his or her skin.

Best sellers for Geremy Rose include Calendula Calming Moisturizer for Dry Skin, made with rich shea and cocoa butters, sweet almond oil, aloe vera and a whole slew of herbal extracts. Their Cucumber Under Eye Treatment is a formulation of fresh botanicals and concentrated extracts to minimize puffiness, dark circles and wrinkles; ingredients include freshly extracted cucumber juice, aloe vera concentrate and shea and cocoa butters. Their Papaya Renewing Moisturizer, rich in skin-softening enzymes, rosewater and a long list of herbal extracts, sounds good enough to eat!

Logona USA, Inc.
554 East Riverside Drive
Ashville, NC 28801
TEL: (800) 648-6654
TEL: (704) 252-1420 — FAX: (704) 252-3570
Website: www.logona.com

German manufacturer Logona Naturkosmetik emerged in the 1970s as a spin-off of the growing environmental movement in Europe. In those early, very "alternative" days, the collectively-organized Logona made very basic products in very basic packaging, which were sold in no-frill Mom-and-Pop stores scattered throughout Germany. Environmental responsibility was broadly defined in this Green movement to encompass both social responsibility and organic agriculture.

Since its early days, Logona has grown into a leading supplier within the German natural product market, offering a comprehensive array of hair, skin and bodycare products. The entire range of Logona products, including the makeups, is made with vegetable oils from organically grown or wildcrafted plants and proven herbal extracts and essential oils, with no synthetic additives of any kind, and no animal testing.

Its products are sold throughout Europe and in the U.S., yet despite its steady growth, the company has remained true to its alternative roots. It continues to streamline its manufacturing processes to achieve better energy efficiency; it still packages minimally, uses organically-grown ingredients whenever possible, and is committed to providing a rewarding, congenial workplace for its employees.

Logona plays an active role in the ongoing process of defining and defending the standards of the natural product marketplace. It works with representatives from other manufacturers, the media and government to maintain the integrity of industry standards, and to develop consensus towards technological changes, such as the current controversy surrounding genetic manipulation in certain raw materials used as ingredients.

Some of Logona's most popular items are their Tinted Daycreams, available in three shades. Because they are German-made, they're formulated with northern European skin tones in mind; however, the Lipstick Pencils are available in a wide range of shades. Logona also makes a full line of eye makeups, including mascara, eyeliner and eye shadows.

Nadina's Cremes, Inc.
3813 Middletown Branch Road
Vienna, MD 21869
TEL: (800) 722-4292 — FAX: (410) 901-1052
Website: www.nadinascremes.com

Jill Nadina Clements literally started Nadina's Cremes in her grandmother's kitchen, and today she has many 100% natural cosmetic products in health food stores all over the U.S. In the early days Jill worked next to her 75-year-old grandmother and their 82-year-old mailman, whose job was to fill the jars with face creams.

"Employing the elderly was not intentional," says Jill. "It just turned out that way, with us giving opportunities to all kinds of people." Today, Nadina's Cremes displays are made by the developmentally challenged, and their creams come in unique jars that are handmade by potters, many of them Native Americans. An earth-friendly company, they recycle everything and use only recycled packaging materials. And, of course, they are also a cruelty-free manufacturer.

"My creams are completely natural," says Jill. "They're made with almond oil, beeswax, aloe vera and essential oils. Sunshine, which is a combination of lemon, orange and bergamot, really gives me a lift. Lavender is more calming, and patchouli, ylang ylang, jasmine and sandalwood are all known aphrodisiacs."

Nadina's Cremes come in 16 natural scents, created from essential oils for a light, delicate fragrance.

Paul Penders Co., Inc.
1340 Commerce St.
Petaluma, CA 94954
TEL: (800) 440-7285 — FAX: (707) 763-5828
Website: http://paulpenders.com.my

Paul Penders started his natural cosmetic company in Holland in the 1960s. During that time the Dutch FDA insisted on testing all cosmetic formulas on animals. When Paul saw the animal testing for himself, he refused to allow his products to be tested and became an impassioned animal rights activist. His company was the very first to advertise it did not test products on animals, and he is to be commended for his courage to speak out against the dangerous and inhumane practice of animal testing.

Paul moved his company to the United States about 15 years ago, and his products are now widely available in health food stores. If you're looking for natural makeups, their eye shadows, blushes and lip colors are about as natural as you're going to find, and they get high ratings from the alternative and natural products experts. His products often incorporate pricey ingredients such as ceramides and alpha-hydroxy acids into all-natural formulas.

Many formulas are based on Penders' exclusive LevensESSENTIE, a combination of 21 herbs the company extracts in-house. Natural Herbal Daytime Moisturizer with Aloe and Lavender for Dry and Sensitive Skin is absorbed very rapidly and leaves the skin soft and smooth. Key ingredients include aloe vera extract, jojoba oil, rice bran wax, vegetable glycerine and essential fatty acids (from flax seeds). In his extensive line of color cosmetics, only pure, natural pigments of iron oxides, carmine and titanium dioxide are used.

Rainbow Research Corporation
170 Wilbur Place
Bohemia, NY 11716
TEL: (800) 722-9595 — FAX: (631) 589-4687
Website: http://www.rainbowresearch.com

Rainbow Research offers natural alternatives to synthetic hair dyes, and provides ways to color your hair naturally, without using highly toxic, often carcinogenic chemicals found in most hair colors. Brown, black, brunette and red permanent and semi-permanent synthetic hair dyes are particularly dangerous; they have been linked to non-Hodgkin's lymphoma, leukemia, multiple myeloma and Hodgkin's disease, and there is also a possible connection to breast cancer. Henna colors are your safest choice, and Rainbow Research Henna comes in a variety of shades to cover grey hair, pick up natural highlights or change your hair color to give you a whole new look.

Rainbow Research was founded in 1976 as a cruelty-free company, and since the very beginning has chosen not to use animal products in any of its formulas. Their philosophy is simple—use the best natural herbal ingredients available, stay away from unnecessary chemicals, and always tell the truth in advertising. Their products are made in small batches to keep their quality high.

Weleda, Inc.
P. O. Box 249
Congers, NY 10920
TEL: (800) 241-1030
TEL: (914) 268-8599 — FAX: (914) 268-8574
Website: www.weleda.com

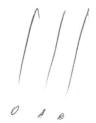

Founded in Switzerland in 1921 by a group of physicians working with Drs. Rudolf Steiner and Ita Wegman, Weleda is a company engaged in the service of anthroposophical medicine, an innovative approach to health care. In choosing the name Weleda, Dr. Steiner honored the ancient tradition of Celtic women healers. Today Weleda is a leading brand for natural medicines and personal care products.

The American branch of the company was started in Manhattan in 1931, and now resides in the historic New York Hudson River Valley. Weleda manufactures and imports high quality, natural personal care products, including shampoos, toothpastes, skin creams, massage oils, deodorants soaps and baby care products. They are distributed directly to health food stores and pharmacies, or are available through mail order.

The chief source of ingredients used in Weleda products is plants. Many of them are organically or biodynamically grown in their own gardens or harvested in the wild in their natural habitats. Naturally occurring minerals such as chalk, clay and silica are also used. The only animal products used in Weleda Body Care preparations are lanolin (from sheep's wool) and beeswax. Their ingredients go through a variety of manufacturing processes, some of which are unique to Weleda. No synthetic preservatives or chemicals are ever used.

Arnica Body and Massage Oil is one top product from this natural company. Peanut and olive oil are the carrying agents for arnica extract, birch leaf extract, rosemary oil and lavender oil. Packaged in a clear glass bottle and an attractive orange and yellow box, this oil is deliciously pungent, a welcome respite after a hard day of hiking or a vigorous workout. Weleda Diaper Care contains 12% zinc oxide as its active ingredient to help prevent and control diaper rash. Almond oil, saponified beeswax, plus extracts of calendula and camomile flowers help soothe and moisturize baby's delicate skin. Their all-natural Sage Deodorant combines grain alcohol with lemon juice, vegetable glycerine and sage oil.

VIII

Resources

Acacia (Gum Arabic) (Spray Dried)
Delamo Chemicals
535 W. 152nd St.
Gardena, CA 90248
310-532-9214

Almond Meal
Look for certified organic almonds in the bulk section of your local
health food store.

Aloe Vera
Aubrey Organics®
4419 N. Manhattan Ave.
Tampa, FL 33614
1-800-282-7394

Lily of the Desert
1887 Greesling Rd.
Denton, TX 76208
940-566-9914

Amino Acids - Max
Country Life Vitamins
101 Corporate Dr.
Hauppauge, NY 11788-2021
1-800-645-5768

Solgar Vitamin & Herb Company
500 Willow Tree Rd.
Leonia, NJ 07605-2232
1-800-645-2246

Angelica Eau de Cologne
Aubrey Organics®
4419 N. Manhattan Ave.
Tampa, FL 33614
1-800-282-7394

Arnica Oil
Aura Cacia
P.O. Box 311
Norway, Iowa 52318
1-800-437-3301

Frontier Cooperative Herbs
2990 Wilderness Pl. (Suite 200)
Boulder, CO 80301
1-800-669-3275

Gaia Herbs, Inc.
108 Island Ford Rd.
Brevard, NC 28712-9730
1-800-831-7780

Avocado Oil
Frontier Cooperative Herbs
2990 Wilderness Pl. (Suite 200)
Boulder, CO 80301
1-800-669-3275

Baking Soda
Available in supermarkets, drug stores and health food stores.

Bentonite Clay
Rainbow Research Corp.
170 Wilbur Pl.
Bohemia, NY 11716-2416
1-800-722-9595

Aztec Secret Health & Beauty
P.O. Box 841
Pahrump, NV 89041
775-727-8351

Bilberry Extract
Gaia Herbs, Inc.
108 Island Ford Rd.
Brevard, NC 28712-9730
1-800-831-7780

Frontier Cooperative Herbs
2990 Wilderness Pl. (Suite 200)
Boulder, CO 80301
1-800-669-3275

Biotin
TwinLab
2120 Smithtown Ave.
Ronkonkoma, NY 11779-7357
631-467-3140

Black Currant Oil
Nutriceutical Corp. Soloray
P.O. Box 681869
Park City, Utah 84068-1869
435-655-6070

Blue Camomile Oil
Aroma Véra
P.O. 3609
Culver City, CA 90231

Blue Green Algae
Klamath Algae Products, Inc.
P.O. Box 1792
Klamath Falls, OR 97601-0102
541-884-2389

Earthrise
424 Payran St.
Petaluma, CA 94952-5903
707-778-9078

Borage Oil
Barleans Organic Oils
4936 Lake Terrell Rd.
Ferndale, WA 98248-9014
1-800-445-3529

Omega Nutrition USA Inc.
6515 Aldrich Rd.
Bellingham, WA 98226
800-661-3529

Bran
Arrowhead Mills
P.O. Box 2059
Hereford, TX 79045-2059
806-364-0730

Calamine & Aloe Lotion (CALAL)
Aubrey Organics®
4419 N. Manhattan Ave.
Tampa, FL 33614
1-800-282-7394

Calendula Oil

Aura Cacia
P.O. Box 311
Norway, Iowa 52318
1-800-437-3301

Frontier Cooperative Herbs
2990 Wilderness Pl. (Suite 200)
Boulder, CO 80301
1-800-669-3275

Camomile Oil (Golden)

Aura Cacia
P.O. Box 311
Norway, Iowa 52318
1-800-437-3301

Frontier Cooperative Herbs
2990 Wilderness Pl. (Suite 200)
Boulder, CO 80301
1-800-669-3275

Gaia Herbs, Inc.
108 Island Ford Rd.
Brevard, NC 28712-9730
1-800-831-7780

Camphor Oil

Aura Cacia
P.O. Box 311
Norway, Iowa 52318
1-800-437-3301

Frontier Cooperative Herbs
2990 Wilderness Pl. (Suite 200)
Boulder, CO 80301
1-800-669-3275

Carrot Seed Oil

Aura Cacia
P.O. Box 311
Norway, Iowa 52318
1-800-437-3301

Frontier Cooperative Herbs
2990 Wilderness Pl. (Suite 200)
Boulder, CO 80301
1-800-669-3275

Castile Soap
Dr. Bronner's All-One God's Faith, Inc.
PO Box 28
Escondido, CA 92033-0028
760-743-2211

Castor Oil
Heritage (Edgar Cayce) Products
P.O. Box 444
Virginia Beach, VA 23458
1-800-862-2923

Cayenne Pepper Oil
Aura Cacia
P.O. Box 311
Norway, Iowa 52318
1-800-437-3301

Frontier Cooperative Herbs
2990 Wilderness Pl. (Suite 200)
Boulder, CO 80301
1-800-669-3275

Cedarwood Oil
Tisserand
E. Newtown Rd.
Hove, E. Sussex
England BN37BA
011-44-127-332-5666

Aura Cacia
P.O. Box 311
Norway, Iowa 52318
1-800-437-3301

Clay
Rainbow Research Corp.
170 Wilbur Pl.
Bohemia, NY 11716-2416
1-800-722-9595

Aztec Secret Health & Beauty
P.O. Box 841; 951 Wilson
Pahrump, NV 89041
775-727-8351

Clay (Green and Red Moroccan Clays)

NOW
395 S. Glen Ellyn Rd.
Bloomingdale, IL 60108
1-800-999-8069

Cocoa Butter

Aura Cacia
P.O. Box 311
Norway, Iowa 52318
1-800-437-3301

Frontier Cooperative Herbs
2990 Wilderness Pl. (Suite 200)
Boulder, CO 80301
1-800-669-3275

Coconut Oil

Spectrum Naturals Inc.
133 Copeland St.
Pataluma, CA 94952-3181
707-778-8900

Frontier Cooperative Herbs
2990 Wilderness Pl. (Suite 200)
Boulder, CO 80301
1-800-669-3275

Cod Liver Oil

TwinLab
2120 Smithtown Ave.
Ronkonkoma, NY 11779-7357
631-467-3140

Country Life Vitamins
101 Corporate Dr.
Hauppauge, NY 11788-2021
1-800-645-5768

Collagen Liquid Protein
TwinLab
2120 Smithtown Ave.
Ronkonkoma, NY 11779-7357
631-467-3140

Comfrey Extract
Herbs of Light, Inc.
PO Box 1648
High Springs, FL 32655
1-800-313-3001

Cornmeal
Available at your grocery store or health food store. Choose organic whenever possible.

Cypress Oil
Tisserand
E. Newtown Rd.
Hove, E. Sussex
England BN37BA
011-44-127-332-5666

Aura Cacia
P.O. Box 311
Norway, Iowa 52318
1-800-437-3301

Essential Fatty Acids
Udo's Oil
Designing Health, Inc.
28310 Avenue Crocker (Suite G)
Valencia, CA 91355-3962
1-800-774-7387

Barleans Organic Oils
4936 Lake Terrell Rd.
Ferndale, WA 98248-9014
1-800-445-3529

Omega Nutrition USA, Inc.
5373 Guide Meridan Rd.
Cascade Business Park
Bellingham, WA 98226-9740

Essential Oils
Aura Cacia
P.O. Box 311
Norway, Iowa 52318
1-800-437-3301

Frontier Cooperative Herbs
2990 Wilderness Pl. (Suite 200)
Boulder, CO 80301
1-800-669-3275

Eucalyptus Oil
Aura Cacia
P.O. Box 311
Norway, Iowa 52318
1-800-437-3301

Frontier Cooperative Herbs
2990 Wilderness Pl. (Suite 200)
Boulder, CO 80301
1-800-669-3275

Evening Primrose Oil
Aubrey Organics®
4419 N. Manhattan Ave.
Tampa, FL 33614
1-800-282-7394

Five Grain Cereal
Available in health food stores.

Flaxseed Oil
Barleans Organic Oils
4936 Lake Terrell Rd.
Ferndale, WA 98248-9014
1-800-445-3529

Arrowhead Mills
P.O. Box 2059
Hereford, TX 79045-2059
806-364-0730

Ginger Oil
Aura Cacia
P.O. Box 311
Norway, Iowa 52318
1-800-437-3301

Frontier Cooperative Herbs
2990 Wilderness Pl. (Suite 200)
Boulder, CO 80301
1-800-669-3275

Gaia Herbs, Inc.
108 Island Ford Rd.
Brevard, NC 28712-9730
1-800-831-7780

Ginger Root Extract
Gaia Herbs, Inc.
108 Island Ford Rd.
Brevard, NC 28712-9730
1-800-831-7780

Grain Alcohol, Natural (76.5% ALC/VOL, 150 Proof)
If you are unable to obtain natural grain alcohol from your local wine and
spirits store, you may use a high grade (triple distilled) vodka in its place.

Grapefruit Oil (Not Grapefruit Seed Oil)
Aura Cacia
P.O. Box 311
Norway, Iowa 52318
1-800-437-3301

Frontier Cooperative Herbs
2990 Wilderness Pl. (Suite 200)
Boulder, CO 80301
1-800-669-3275

Gaia Herbs, Inc.
108 Island Ford Rd.
Brevard, NC 28712-9730
1-800-831-7780

Grapefruit Seed Extract
Nutribiotic
133 Copeland St. (Suite C)
Petaluma, CA 94952-3181
707-769-2266

Green Clay (French)
Rainbow Research Corp.
170 Wilbur Pl.
Bohemia, NY 11716-2416
1-800-722-9595

Now Foods
550 Mitchell Rd.
Glendale Heights, IL 60139-2581
1-800-999-8069

Green Kamut®
Green Kamut Corp.
1542 Sea Bright Ave.
Long Beach, CA 90813
1-800-452-6884

Green Magma®
Frontier Cooperative Herbs
2990 Wilderness Pl. (Suite 200)
Boulder, CO 80301
1-800-669-3275

Green Tea Extract
Aura Cacia
P.O. Box 311
Norway, Iowa 52318
1-800-437-3301

Frontier Cooperative Herbs
2990 Wilderness Pl. (Suite 200)
Boulder, CO 80301
1-800-669-3275

Gaia Herbs, Inc.
108 Island Ford Rd.
Brevard, NC 28712-9730
1-800-831-7780

244

Eden Foods
701 Tecumseh Road
Clinton, MI 49236-9599
517-456-7424

Green Tea Leaves
Select Herb Tea Co.
1351 Marlhardt Ave.
Oxnard, CA 93030
888-273-3532

Gum Arabic (also see Acacia)
Available in the bulk foods section of your health food store.

Henna
Rainbow Research Corp.
170 Wilbur Pl.
Bohemia, NY 11716-2416
1-800-722-9595

Herbal Liquid Body Soap
Aubrey Organics®
4419 N. Manhattan Ave.
Tampa, FL 33614
1-800-282-7394

Horse Chestnut
Gaia Herbs, Inc.
108 Island Ford Rd.
Brevard, NC 28712-9730
1-800-831-7780

Zand Herbal Formulas
1722 14th St. (Suite 230)
Boulder, CO 80302
1-800-800-0405

Horsetail (Alcohol-Free)
Nature's Answer, Inc.
75 Commerce Dr.
Hauppauge, NY 11788
1-800-439-2324

(You may use horsetail from the following sources if you let the alcohol evaporate first.)

Herbs of Light, Inc.
PO Box 1648
High Springs, FL 32655
1-800-313-3001

Gaia Herbs, Inc.
108 Island Ford Rd.
Brevard, NC 28712-9730
1-800-831-7780

Jojoba Butter
Frontier Cooperative Herbs
2990 Wilderness Pl. (Suite 200)
Boulder, CO 80301
1-800-669-3275

Jojoba Oil (Organic)
Aubrey Organics®
4419 N. Manhattan Ave.
Tampa, FL 33614
1-800-282-7394

Kava Kava
Gaia Herbs, Inc.
108 Island Ford Rd.
Brevard, NC 28712-9730
1-800-831-7780

Pioneer Nutritional Formulas, Inc.
304 Shelburne Center Rd.
Shelburne Falls, MA 01370-9779
1-800-458-8483

Kelp
Alternatives
P.O. Box 91
Buffalo, NY 14207-0091
1-800-987-7100

Lavender Oil
Tisserand
E. Newtown Rd.
Hove, E. Sussex
England BN37BA
011-44-1273-332-5666

Gaia Herbs, Inc.
108 Island Ford Rd.
Brevard, NC 28712-9730
1-800-831-7780

Aura Cacia
P.O. Box 311
Norway, Iowa 52318
1-800-437-3301

L-Cystine
Country Life Vitamins
101 Corporate Dr.
Hauppauge, NY 11788-2021
1-800-645-5768

Lecithin (Oil)
Country Life Vitamins
101 Corporate Dr.
Hauppauge, NY 11788-2021
1-800-645-5768

Solgar Vitamin & Herb Company
500 Willow Tree Rd.
Leonia, NJ 07605-2232
1-800-645-2246

Lemon Blossom Body Splash
Aubrey Organics®
4419 N. Manhattan Ave.
Tampa, FL 33614
1-800-282-7394

Lemon Peel Oil
Aura Cacia
P.O. Box 311
Norway, Iowa 52318
1-800-437-3301

Frontier Cooperative Herbs
2990 Wilderness Pl. (Suite 200)
Boulder, CO 80301
1-800-669-3275

Licorice Root
Gaia Herbs, Inc.
108 Island Ford Rd.
Brevard, NC 28712-9730
1-800-831-7780

Pioneer Nutritional Formulas, Inc.
304 Shelburne Center Rd.
Shelburne Falls, MA 01370-9779
1-800-458-8483

Loofa
Body Tools
16 Pamaron Way (Suite C)
Novato, CA 94949-6217
1-800-845-6202

Milk Thistle Extract
Gaia Herbs, Inc.
108 Island Ford Rd.
Brevard, NC 28712-9730
1-800-831-7780

Pioneer Nutritional Formulas, Inc.
304 Shelburne Center Rd.
Shelburne Falls, MA 01370-9779
1-800-458-8483

Musk Splash
Aubrey Organics®
4419 N. Manhattan Ave.
Tampa, FL 33614
1-800-282-7394

Neem Oil
Neem Aura Naturals
10105 NW 156th Ave.
Alachua, FL 32615-5045
352-375-2503

Auromere Ayurvedic Imports
2621 W. US Hwy. 12
Lodi, CA 95242-9200
1-800-735-4691

Nettle
Available at bulk herb section of your health food store.

Oats (Organic)
Prairie Mills Co.
P.O. Box 820
Wayzata, MN 55391-0820
763-473-9407

Oregano Oil (Wild Marjoram)
North American Herb and Spice Company
P.O. Box 4885
Buffalo Grove, IL 60089
1-800-243-5242

Solgar Vitamin & Herb Company
500 Willow Tree Rd.
Leonia, NJ 07605-2232
1-800-645-2246

Bluebonnet Nutrition Corp.
12915 Dairy Ashford
Sugarland, TX 77478
281-240-3332

PABA
Country Life Vitamins
101 Corporate Dr.
Hauppauge, NY 11788-2021
1-800-645-5768

Solgar Vitamin & Herb Company
500 Willow Tree Rd.
Leonia, NJ 07605-2232
1-800-645-2246

Palm Kernel Oil
Spectrum Naturals Inc.
133 Copeland St.
Petaluma, CA 94952-3181
707-778-8900

Hain Food Group
50 Charles Linbergh Blvd. (Suite 100)
Uniondale, NY 11553-3600
516-237-6200

Pantothenic Acid (Panthenol)
Country Life Vitamins
101 Corporate Dr.
Hauppauge, NY 11788-2021
1-800-645-5768

Solgar Vitamin & Herb Company
500 Willow Tree Rd.
Leonia, NJ 07605-2232
1-800-645-2246

Papain
Adolph's Tenderizer Original (Unseasoned)
800 Sylvan Ave.
Angelwood Cliffs, NJ 07632
1-800-328-7248
(May also be available in the bulk herb section of your heath food store.)

Pectin (Liquid)
Certo Liquid Fruit Pectin
Kraft General Foods, Inc.
1 Kraft Court
Glenview, IL 60025
1-800-437-3284

Pectin (Powder)
Sure-Jel
Kraft General Foods, Inc.
Box SJ
White Plains, NY 10625
1-800-437-3284

Peppermint Oil
Aura Cacia
P.O. Box 311
Norway, Iowa 52318
1-800-437-3301

Frontier Cooperative Herbs
2990 Wilderness Pl. (Suite 200)
Boulder, CO 80301
1-800-669-3275

Gaia Herbs, Inc.
108 Island Ford Rd.
Brevard, NC 28712-9730
1-800-831-7780

Perrier Sparkling Mineral Water®
Available in supermarkets and health food stores.

Pine Oil
Aura Cacia
P.O. Box 311
Norway, Iowa 52318
1-800-437-3301

ProGreens®
Nutricology
30806 Santana St.
Hayward, CA 94544
510-487-8526

Psyllium Husk Powder
Yerba Prima, Inc.
740 Jefferson Ave.
Ashland, OR 95720-3743
541-488-2228

(Also available in the bulk food section of your health food store.)

Pycnogenol
Country Life Vitamins
101 Corporate Dr.
Hauppauge, NY 11788-2021
1-800-645-5768

Solgar Vitamin & Herb Company
500 Willow Tree Rd.
Leonia, NJ 07605-2232
1-800-645-2246

Rice Cream (Brown)
Erewhon Organic Brown Rice Cream
U.S. Mills, Inc.
200 Reservoir St.
Needham, MA 02494
781-444-0440

Rice Oil
Spectrum Naturals Inc.
133 Copeland St.
Petaluma, CA 94952-3181
707-778-8900

Rice Powder
Westbrae/Little Bear Natural Foods
1065 E. Walnut St.
Carson, CA 90746-1316
310-886-8200

Rosa Mosqueta® Rose Hip Seed Oil
Aubrey Organics®
4419 N. Manhattan Ave.
Tampa, FL 33614
1-800-282-7394

Rosemary Oil
Aura Cacia
P.O. Box 311
Norway, Iowa 52318
1-800-437-3301

Gaia Herbs, Inc.
108 Island Ford Rd.
Brevard, NC 28712-9730
1-800-831-7780

Rosewater
Frontier Cooperative Herbs
2990 Wilderness Pl. (Suite 200)
Boulder, CO 80301
1-800-669-3275
(Also Check in your local pharmacy or in the specialty supermarket.)

Rose Oil
Aura Cacia
P.O. Box 311
Norway, Iowa 52318
1-800-437-3301

Frontier Cooperative Herbs
2990 Wilderness Pl. (Suite 200)
Boulder, CO 80301
1-800-669-3275

Royal Jelly
Y.S. Organic Bee Farms
RR1 Box 91A
Sheridan, IL 60551-9629
815-496-9416

Sage Oil
Aura Cacia
P.O. Box 311
Norway, Iowa 52318
1-800-437-3301

Gaia Herbs, Inc.
108 Island Ford Rd.
Brevard, NC 28712-9730
1-800-831-7780

Sandalwood Oil
Aura Cacia
P.O. Box 311
Norway, Iowa 52318
1-800-437-3301

Frontier Cooperative Herbs
2990 Wilderness Pl. (Suite 200)
Boulder, CO 80301
1-800-669-3275

Gaia Herbs, Inc.
108 Island Ford Rd.
Brevard, NC 28712-9730
1-800-831-7780

Seasoap
Aubrey Organics®
4419 N. Manhattan Ave.
Tampa, FL 33614
1-800-282-7394

Shea Butter
Frontier Cooperative Herbs
2990 Wilderness Pl. (Suite 200)
Boulder, CO 80301
1-800-669-3275

Karite-One
Mode de Vie, CA 91710
1-800-474-4304

Selenium
Country Life Vitamins
101 Corporate Dr.
Hauppauge, NY 11788-2021
1-800-645-5768

Solgar Vitamin & Herb Company
500 Willow Tree Rd.
Leonia, NJ 07605-2232
1-800-645-2246

Soybean Oil
Spectrum Naturals Inc.
133 Copeland St.
Pataluma, CA 94952-3181
707-778-8900

Spearmint Oil
Aura Cacia
P.O. Box 311
Norway, Iowa 52318
1-800-437-3301

Frontier Cooperative Herbs
2990 Wilderness Pl. (Suite 200)
Boulder, CO 80301
1-800-669-3275

Gaia Herbs, Inc.
108 Island Ford Rd.
Brevard, NC 28712-9730
1-800-831-7780

St. John's Wort Oil
Aura Cacia
P.O. Box 311
Norway, Iowa 52318
1-800-437-3301

Frontier Cooperative Herbs
2990 Wilderness Pl. (Suite 200)
Boulder, CO 80301
1-800-669-3275

Gaia Herbs, Inc.
108 Island Ford Rd.
Brevard, NC 28712-9730
1-800-831-7780

Sulfur (Powder)
Available in drug stores and pharmacies

Tea Tree Oil
Dessert Essence
9700 Topanga Canyon Blvd.
Chatsworth, CT 91311
516-231-1031

Aura Cacia
P.O. Box 311
Norway, Iowa 52318
1-800-437-3301

Tofu
Mori-Nu
2050 W. 190th St. (Suite 110)
Torrance, CA 90504-6230
1-800-669-8638

VitaSoy
400 Oyster Point Blvd. (Suite 201)
S. San Francisco, CA 94080-1904
1-800-848-2769

Eden Foods, Inc.
701 Tecumseh Rd.
Clinton, MI 49236-9599
517-456-7424

Tomato Paste
Muir Glen Organic Tomato Products
PO Box 200
Minneapolis, MN
1-800-832-6345

Tragacanth Gum
Available in the bulk food section of your health food store.

Vegetable Glycerine
Rainbow Research Corp.
170 Wilbur Pl.
Bohemia, NY 11716-2416
1-800-722-9595

(Also check in your local pharmacy or in the specialty supermarket.)

Vegetable Protein
Naturade, Inc.
14370 Myford Rd. (Suite 100)
Irvine, CA 92606
714-573-4800

Vitamin B-Complex
Country Life Vitamins
101 Corporate Dr.
Hauppauge, NY 11788-2021
1-800-645-5768

Solgar Vitamin & Herb Company
500 Willow Tree Rd.
Leonia, NJ 07605-2232
1-800-645-2246

Vitamin C (Liquid)
TwinLab
2120 Smithtown Ave.
Ronkonkoma, NY 11779-7357
631-467-3140

Vitamin C (Powdered)
Look for pure, powdered ascorbic acid.

Country Life Vitamins
101 Corporate Dr.
Hauppauge, NY 11788-2021
1-800-645-5768

Solgar Vitamin & Herb Company
500 Willow Tree Rd.
Leonia, NJ 07605-2232
1-800-645-2246

Bluebonnet Nutrition Corp.
12503 Exchange Drive
Stafford, TX 77477-3607
1-800-680-8866

Vitamin E (Oil)
Viobin USA
226 W. Livingston St.
Monticello, IL 61856-1632
217-762-2561

Wheat Germ Oil
Spectrum Naturals Inc.
133 Copeland St.
Pataluma, CA 94952-3181
701-778-8900

Frontier Cooperative Herbs
P.O. 299
Norway, IA 52318-0299
1-800-669-3275

White Camellia Oil
Aubrey Organics®
4419 N. Manhattan Ave.
Tampa, FL 33614
1-800-282-7394

Wintergreen Oil
Aura Cacia
P.O. Box 311
Norway, Iowa 52318
1-800-437-3301

Frontier Cooperative Herbs
2990 Wilderness Pl. (Suite 200)
Boulder, CO 80301
1-800-669-3275

Gaia Herbs, Inc.
108 Island Ford Rd.
Brevard, NC 28712-9730
1-800-831-7780

Witch Hazel
Available in most health food stores and local pharmacies.

Yogurt
Horizon Organic Dairy
6311 Horizon Ln.
Longmont, CO 80503
303-530-2711

Stoneyfield Farm Yogurt
10 Burton Dr.
Londerderry, NH 03053-7436
603-437-3935

Yucca Root Extract
Gaia Herbs, Inc.
108 Island Ford Rd.
Brevard, NC 28712-9730
1-800-831-7780

Pioneer Nutritional Formulas, Inc.
304 Shelburne Center Rd.
Shelburne Falls, MA 01370-9779
1-800-458-8483

Yucca and Burdock Extract
TwinLab
2120 Smithtown Ave.
Ronkonkoma, NY 11779-7357
631-467-3140

BIBLIOGRAPHY

Alive Research Group. *Encyclopedia of Natural Healing*. Burnaby, BC, Canada: Alive Books, 1997.

Balin, Arthur K., M.D. Ph.D., Loretta Pratt Balin, M.D., and Marietta Whittlesey. *The Life of the Skin: What it Hides, What it Reveals and How it Communicates*. New York: Bantam, 1997.

"Being Beautiful: Deciding for Yourself. Selected Readings." Washington, D, C. Center for the Study of Responsive Law, 1985.

Begoun, Paula. *Don't Go to the Cosmetics Counter Without Me: An Eye-Opening Guide to Brand-Name Cosmetics*. Seattle, WA: Beginning Press, 1996.

Broadhurst, C. Leigh, Ph.D. *The Evolutionary Diet: A Plan for Weight Balance and Optimum Health*. Omega Nutrition, 1997.

Bunney, Sarah. *The Illustrated Encyclopedia of Herbs*. New York, Dorset Press, 1984.

Castleman, Michael. *Nature's Cures: From Acupressure and Aromatherapy to Walking and Yoga, The Ultimate Guide to the Best Scientifically Proven, Drug-Free Healing Methods*. Emmaus, PA: Rodale Press, 1996.

Colborn, Theo, Dianne Dumanoski, and John Peterson Myers. *Our Stolen Future*. New York: Penguin, 1996.

Cooksley, Valerie Gennari. *Aromatherapy: A Lifetime Guide to Healing with Essential Oils*. Englewod Cliffs, NJ: Prentice Hall, 1996.

Diamond, Nina L. *Purify Your Body*. New York: Crown Trade Paperbacks, 1996

Duke, James A., Ph.D. *The Green Pharmacy*, Emmaus, PA: Rodale Press, 1997.

Erasmus, Udo. *Fats That Heal, Fats That Kill*. Burnaby, BC, Canada: Alive Books, 1993.

Grieve, M. *A Modern Herbal*. (In Two Volumes), New York, NY: Dover Publications, New York, N.Y., 1971.

Hampton, Aubrey. *Natural Organic Hair and Skin Care*. Tampa, FL: Organica Press, 1987.

Hampton, Aubrey. *What's in Your Cosmetics? A Complete Consumer's Guide to Natural and Synthetic Ingredients.* Tucson, AZ: Odonian Press, 1995.

Lappé, Marc, Ph.D. *The Body's Edge: Our Cultural Obsession with Skin.* New York: Henry Holt and Company, 1996.

Leung, Albert and Steven Foster. *Encyclopedia of Common Natural Ingredients. Used in Foods, Drugs, and Cosmetics.* New York: John Wiley & Sons, 1996.

Prevention Magazine Health Books Editors and the Rodale Center for Women's Health. *Age Erasers for Women.* Emmaus, PA: Rodale Books, 1994.

Pugliese, Peter T., M.D. *Physiology of the Skin.* New York: Allured Publishing System, 1996.

Schwitters, Bert. *OPC in Practice: The Hidden Story of Proanthocyanidins, Nature's Most Powerful and Patented Antioxidant.* Rome, Italy: Alfa Omega Editrice, 1995.

Science Action Coalition. *Consumer's Guide to Cosmetics.* New York: Anchor/ Doubleday, 1980.

Smeh, Nikolaus J. M.S. *Health Risks in Today's Cosmetics: The Handbook for a Lifetime of Healthy Skin and Hair.* Garrisonville, VA: Alliance Publishing, 1994.

Steinman, David and Samuel S. Epstein, M.D. *The Safe Shopper's Bible: A Consumer's Guide to Nontoxic Household Products, Cosmetics and Food.* New York: Macmillan, 1995.

Winter, Ruth. *A Consumer's Dictionary of Cosmetic Ingredients: Complete Information about the Harmful and Desirable Ingredients Found in Men's and Women's Cosmetics.* New York: Crown Publishing, 1989.

Whitaker, Julian, M.D. *Dr. Whitaker's Guide to Natural Healing: America's Leading "Wellness Doctor" Shares His Secrets for Lifelong Health.* Rocklin, CA: Prima Publishing, 1996.

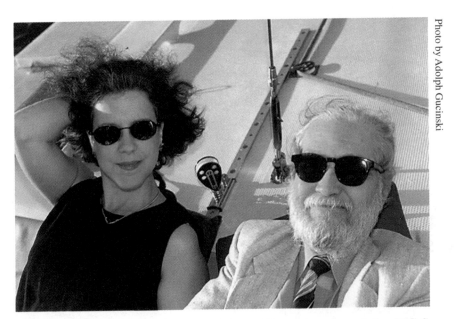

The authors, Susan Hussey and Aubrey Hampton, aboard the U.S.S. FantiSea in the Florida Keys, February 1999.

About the Authors

Aubrey Hampton is the husband of Susan Hussey. He was born in Indiana and educated in New York. He is an organic chemist and phytochemist and has created over 200 natural herbal cosmetics for Aubrey Organics®, a company he founded in 1967, and whose products are sold all over the world. His book, *Natural Organic Hair and Skin Care* (1987, Organica Press) is in its seventh printing and has sold hundreds of thousands of copies. Some of his other books are: *What's in Your Cosmetics* (1995, Odonian Press); *GBS & Company*, a full-length play about the Irish playwright Bernard Shaw (1989, Organica Press), and *Wolf Trilogy* (1991, Organica Press). Aubrey was a magician and ventriloquist in circuses and carnivals as a youth, and is cofounder of The Gorilla Theatre Company. He resides in New York City and Tampa, Florida.

Susan Hussey is the wife of Aubrey Hampton. She was born in Indiana and attended the University of Indiana. She received her graduate degree from the University of South Florida. She was editor of *Natural Organic Hair and Skin Care* (1987, Organica Press) and is also the editor of Organica Press. Susan was a box jumper in carnivals and circuses in her youth. She is cofounder of The Gorilla Theatre, and is a poet and playwright. She resides in New York City and Tampa, Florida.

Index

Arthritis, 78

Art of Aroma Therapy, The, 105

Aspirin (Acetylsalicylic acid), 64

Asthma, 81

Athlete's foot, 108

Aubrey Organics®, 1, 3, 13, 91, 105, 106, 109, 111, 114, 118, 137, 143, 145, 147, 149, 151, 153, 161, 162, 163, 165, 173, 177, 181, 189, 191, 197, 199, 205, 207, 213, 214, 225, 226, 235, 237, 242, 245-248, 252, 253, 257

Aubrey's Facial Flowers Steam Concentrate, 29, 167

Aubrey's Herbal Base, 139, 147, 149, 166, 167

Aubrey's Herbal Facial Astringent, 149

Aubrey's Sparkling Mineral Water Herbal Facial Spray, 31, 165

Aubrey's Tofu Essential Fatty Acid Cream Base, 137

Aura Cacia, 143, 145, 149, 162, 165, 166, 181, 185, 195, 197-199, 201, 205, 235, 238-244, 246, 247, 250, 252, 253, 254, 255, 257

Auromere Ayurvedic Imports, 248

Autumn Harp Inc., 226

Avery, Alexandra, 225

Avicenna, 117

Avocado oil, 94, 105, 119, 236

"Away with You" Herbal Insect Deterrent Spray, 195

Aztec Secret Health & Beauty, 236, 240

B

Baking Soda, 236

Barleans Organic Oils, 137, 162, 163, 207, 237, 241, 242

B-complex vitamins, (see Vitamins, B-complex)

Beeswax, 137, 226, 232

Bentonite clay, 95, 236

Benzoin gum, 95, 139

Beta carotene, 78, 97, 112, 113

Bilberry herb, 95, 236

Bilberry oil, 157

Biodegradable, 223

Bioflavonoids, 123

Biotin, 81, 95, 115, 177, 185-186, 236
    role in dandruff, 181

Birch leaf extract, 232

Birch oil, 64

Black currant, 96, 237

Block, Gladys, Ph.D., 73

Bluebonnet Nutrition Corp., 249, 256

Blue camomile oil, 97, 157, 226, 237

Blue Camomile Shampoo, 226

Blue Green Algae (Microalgae), 97, 112, 113, 151, 183, 185, 186, 237

Blue Green Algae Hair Rescue Mask, 67, 121, 183, 185

Blue Green Algae Hair Rescue Shampoo, 67, 94, 121, 183
Body Shop, 226
Body Tools, 248
Borage oil, 96, 237
Bran, 237
Brazil nut oil, 226
Breast cancer, 77
Broadhurst, C. Leigh, Ph.D., 213-214
Bronner, James, 227
Brushing the Skin, 87
Buccinator muscle, 54
Burdock root, 96, 177, 181
B vitamins, (see Vitamins, B and B-complex)

C

Cade tar, 64
Caffeine, 108
Calamine, 96
Calamine & Aloe Lotion (CALAL), 237
Calcium, 84, 112
Calendula blossoms, 139, 238
Calendula Calming Moisturizer, 228
Calendula extract, 232
Calendula oil, 96, 225
Cameron, Dr. Ewan, 82
Camomile, blue, 96
Camomile flowers, 139
Camomile oil (golden), 97, 232, 238
Camphor oil, 97, 143, 199, 201, 202, 226, 238
Canadian willowherb, 124
Cancer, 73, 76
Candellia wax, 226
Candida albicans, 97, 113, 199
Candidiasis, 106
Capsaicin (cayenne pepper oil), 98, 201, 202, 239
Carbohydrates, 20
Carcinogens, 15
Cardiovascular disease (role of Calcium in), 84
Carmine, 230
Carnauba wax, 226
Carnegie Hall, 165
Carotenoid, 78, 116
Carrey, Jim, 151
Carrot juice, 187
Carrot oil, 97, 123, 238
Carvacrol, 114
Carvajal, Fabiola, M.D., 117
Castile soap, 98, 118, 239

Cystine, 62, 93

D

Dandruff, 61, 63, 92, 110, 121, 181
Dandruff (role of Biotin in), 95
Danhoff, I. E. Ph.D., M.D., 92
DEA (Diethanolamine), 215
Delamo Chemicals, 191, 235
Dermal papilla, 64
Dermatologists, 14
Dermis, 20, 25
Desert Essence, 143, 183, 199, 201, 254
Designing Health Inc., 241
Diabetes, 76, 79
    role of Vitamin C in, 82
Diabetic neuropathy, 81
Diaper rash, 106
Diazolidinyl urea (Germall II), 214
Dibromochloropropane (DBCP), 22
Dickenson Corp., 147, 149, 167
Diet for a Poisoned Planet, 212
Diethanolamine (DEA), 212, 227
Dilantin, 79
DNA (the effect of pesticides on), 77
d-Panthenol, 63, 64
Dr. Bronner's All-One Faith, Inc., 153, 155, 171, 177, 181, 226, 227, 239
Dr. Bronner's Almond Castile Soap, 177, 178
Dr. Bronner's Lavender Castile Soap, 155, 171
Dr. Bronner's Peppermint Castile Soap, 181, 182, 227
Dr. Duke's Hair Saver Rosemary & Sage Shampoo, 181
Dr. Hauschka Cleansing Cream, 228
Dr. Hauschka Cosmetics U.S.A., Inc., 227
Dr. Hauschka Face Lotion, 228
Dr. Hauschka Skin Conditioner, 228
Dr. Hauschka's chemical-free lipsticks, 228
Doctors' Prescription for Healthy Living, The, 212 , 213
Duke, James, Ph. D., 181
Duke, Mark, 42

E

Earthrise Co., 237
Echinacea (Coneflower), 101, 139
E. Coli, 106
Eczema, 64, 77, 80, 83, 109, 205, 208
Eden Foods, 137, 143, 161, 244, 255
Elastin, 21, 25

267

K

L

M

Papyrus Ebers, 92
Para-aminobenzoic acid (PABA), 114, 115, 163, 164
Parkinson's disease, 76
Paul Penders Co., Inc., 230
PCO (procyanidolic oligomers), 86
Peanut oil, 105, 232
Pectin, 115, 250
Pellagra, 78
Peppermint leaves, 153
Peppermint oil, 115, 143, 149, 198, 199, 201, 202, 250
Periodontal disease (and Aloe Vera), 92
Perrier® sparkling mineral water, 116, 165, 250
Pesticides (effect on DNA), 77
Petrochemicals, 13, 101
Petrolatum, 101
Phosphorus, 112, 121
Pine oil, 116, 183, 198, 250
Pioneer Nutritional Formulas, Inc., 145, 198, 246-248, 258
Plerygoid internus muscle, 56
Pliny the Elder, 92, 114
Polyphenols, 107, 116
    In green tea, 86
Polysaccharides, 92
Polyunsaturated fatty acids, 102
Polyunsaturated vegetable oils, 84
Potassium, 85, 121
Prairie Mills Co., 248
Premenstrual syndrome (PMS), 96
    Role of Vitamin E in, 83
Preservatives, 211, 223, 227
ProGreens®, 116, 185, 251
Propyl paraben, 101, 217
Propylene glycol, 216
Prostaglandins, 75
Prostate cancer, 77
Protein metabolism (role of Selenium), 86
Proteins, 93, 113, 155
Psoriasis, 63, 64, 113, 122
Psyllium husks powder, 116, 153, 171, 177, 178, 182, 218, 251
PVP co-polymers, 68, 191, 219
Pycnogenol, 251
Pyridoxine (Vitamin B-6), 80
Pythagoras, 7

Q

Quaternium-15, 212
Quick oats, 116, 153
Quillaya bark, 64
Quince seed, 116

R

Rainbow Research, 151, 230, 236, 239, 243, 244, 255
Rainbow Research Henna, 231, 245
Red Mask Alpha-Hydroxy Fruit Acid Treatment, 95, 157
Relax-R-Bath, 105, 197, 225
Reticulin, 21, 25
Retin-A, 14
Retinoic acid, 122
Riboflavin (Vitamin B-2), 79
Rice bran wax, 230
Rice cream, 116, 251
Rice oil, 251
Rice powder, 218, 251
RNA (ribonucleic acid), 112
Rodale Press, 181
Rosa Mosqueta® & Lavender Herbal Toner, 147
Rosa Mosqueta® Oil, 96, 102, 116, 117, 145, 147, 151, 152, 161-164, 216, 226, 252
Rosa Mosqueta® Rose Hip Moisturizing Cream, 226
Rosa Mosqueta® Super Protein Shampoo, 179
Rosemary, 64, 117, 139, 226
Rosemary & Sage Hair Rinse, 181
Rosemary oil, 143, 149, 181, 185, 195, 197, 198, 232, 252
Rose oil, 118, 252
Rosewater, 117,185, 225, 252
Rothman, Stephen, 22
Royal jelly, 118, 252
Royal Swedish Academy of Sciences, 211
Rutgers State University of New Jersey, 108, 161
Rutin, 123

S

Safe Shopper's Bible, The, 212
Sage, 64, 118, 139, 143, 181, 185, 195, 226, 232, 252
Sage Deodorant, 232
Salicylic acid, 64
Salmonella, 106
Sandalwood oil, 118, 253
Sarsaparilla root, 64

T

U

V